Practical and Postmortem Record Book of

Forensic Medicine and Toxicology

Name of the Student ______________________

College/Institute ______________________

Class Roll No. ______________ *Session/Year* ______________

University Roll No. ______________________

Practical and Postmortem Record Book of
Forensic Medicine and Toxicology

Gautam Biswas MD
Professor and Head
Department of Forensic Medicine and Toxicology
Dayanand Medical College and Hospital
Ludhiana, Punjab, India

Forewords

Narinder K Aggarwal
Tapas K Bose

JAYPEE

JAYPEE BROTHERS MEDICAL PUBLISHERS
The Health Sciences Publisher
New Delhi | London

JAYPEE Jaypee Brothers Medical Publishers (P) Ltd.

Headquarters

EMCA House
23/23-B, Ansari Road, Daryaganj
New Delhi 110 002, India
Landline: +91-11-23272143,
+91-11-23272703+91-11-23282021,
+91-11-23245672
E-mail: jaypee@jaypeebrothers.com

Corporate Office
Jaypee Brothers Medical Publishers (P) Ltd.
4838/24, Ansari Road, Daryaganj
New Delhi 110 002, India
Phone: +91-11-43574357
Fax: +91-11-43574314
E-mail: jaypee@jaypeebrothers.com

Overseas Off ce
JP Medical Ltd.
83, Victoria Street, London
SW1H 0HW (UK)
Phone: +44-20 3170 8910
E-mail: info@jpmedpub.com

EU GPSR Authorised Representative
Logos Europe, 9 rue Nicolas Poussin
17000, La Rochelle, France
Phone: +33 (0) 6 67 93 73 78
E-mail: Contact@logoseurope.eu

Website: www.jaypeebrothers.com
Website: www.jaypeedigital.com

Inquiries for bulk sales may be solicited at: jaypee@jaypeebrothers.com

Practical and Postmortem Record Book of Forensic Medicine and Toxicology

First Edition: 2016

Reprint: **2024, 2025**

ISBN 978-93-5250-155-7

Printed in India

Dedicated

to

My Son Gaurav

&

All my students — Past, Present and Future

'Tell me and I'll forget. Show me and I'll remember. Involve me and I'll understand'

—Confucius

Foreword

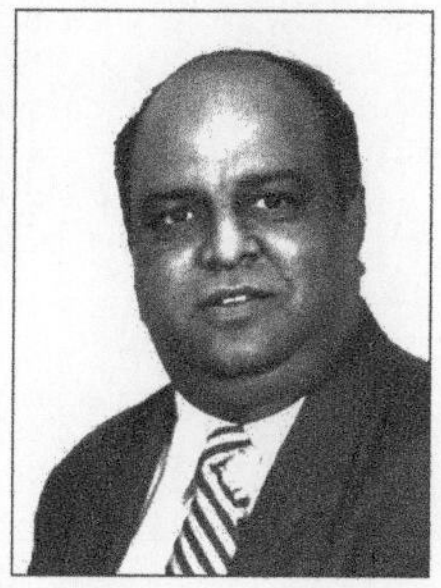

Watching his students excel in their field is one of the most rewarding moments for a teacher. Writing this piece makes me joyous, honored and proud at the same time. Gautam was a student of mine during his graduation. He has authored many immensely popular books in the field of Forensic Medicine and Toxicology, but this *Practical and Postmortem Record Book of Forensic Medicine and Toxicology* was the need of the hour. The hard work done by him in bringing out this book is highly commendable. The book is quite comprehensive in the undergraduate syllabus and will also be helpful to the medical practitioners in their day-to-day practice. It contains all types of proforma from issue of medical certificates to examination of all types of hypothetical medicolegal cases, and also gives an in-depth knowledge of the subject in addition to it.

Clinical forensic medicine is the highlight of this book. Details about the examination of an individual for the estimation of age, examination of a survivor in sexual assault, examination of an accused in sexual assault, examination of a case of alleged impotence, and examination of a patient in the cases of poisoning and drunkenness are given in the book. Detailed examination of a case of recent delivery and psychiatric examination of a person are also given.

A new innovative concept/exercise called *Project* has been added in this book. It will help the students learn the method of writing case reports. They are exposed to various parts of paper-writing, which includes references. Specific exercises like determination of age from X-rays, examination of skeletal remains, and museum specimens and instruments used for autopsy have been described properly.

I wish him great success and a bright future ahead. I am sure this record book will be very useful to the undergraduate students.

Narinder K Aggarwal
MD MNAMS FIAMLE FICFMT WHO Fellow
Professor and Head
Department of Forensic Medicine and Toxicology
University College of Medical Sciences
Delhi, India
Formerly
Head
Department of Forensic Medicine and Toxicology
University of Delhi
Delhi, India

Foreword

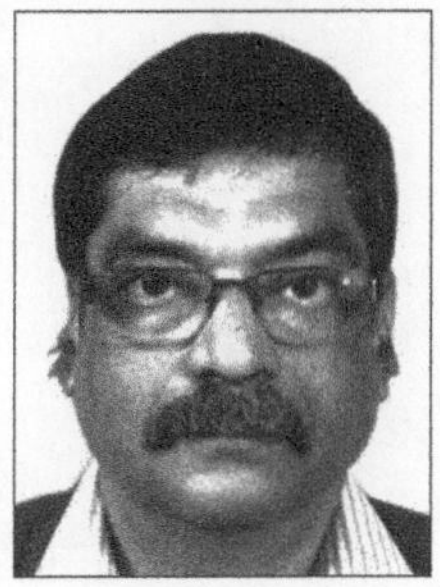

The writer of this *vade mecum* (etymology: Latin – 'go with me' – a book for ready reference) has undertaken the task of preparation of this volume primarily for the practical in the second professional MBBS course. A society has a justifiable demand to expect an optimum service from a doctor not only in healthcare but also to participate in the disbursement of justice pertaining not only to the offences involving human body but again to solve civil litigations, like age or sex estimation. Otherwise the law will be obstructed in its own flow. Unfortunately, though Forensic Medicine is a science which teaches the application of every branch of medical knowledge for the purpose of law and actually a practical subject, the practical part is most neglected and there is till now no standard guidebook for the students in practical forensic medicine as well as no uniformity in practical teaching in different institutions, and the practicals become a less important job, mostly a recapitulation of the theory like a vestigial organ.

After having the basic qualification, the students become doctors and are exposed to the reality of the cases, consent, dying declarations, litigations, police reporting, sexual assaults, CPA, etc. Unless they have the sound knowledge in practicals, they enter into a puzzle with no answer.

This *Practical and Postmortem Record Book of Forensic Medicine and Toxicology* is informative, and, in a systematic way, it has touched all the necessities of an undergraduate student not merely to pass the examination but also as a guidebook for future and has done the excellent job of making the students interested to learn, and promote fun and joy of learning. I am sure this book will find a place in the desks of all the students, breaking the concept of collegewise practical books to uniformity throughout the national level and useful to all the users.

I wish every success to the pioneer endeavor of my good old friend.

Tapas K Bose
Professor and Head
Department of Forensic Medicine and Toxicology
Nilratan Sarkar Medical College
Kolkata, West Bengal, India
Member Secretary, Board of Studies in UG and PG, Forensic Medicine
West Bengal University of Health Sciences
Council Member, IAFM (2013–2016), Indian Academy of Forensic Sciences
Advisor
Indian Society of Toxicology

Preface

It gives me immense pleasure to present this *Practical and Postmortem Record Book of Forensic Medicine and Toxicology* to the undergraduate students. Conventionally, the students are required to fill up the practical record book as a part of their teaching in Forensic Medicine and Toxicology. Although there are guidelines for recording medicolegal cases, there is no agreed system for recording the information in these files. These files are outdated and incomplete in many aspects since there is no standardization of practicals. The way students report their findings varies in different institutes and in different states. The inconsistencies which are there during the learning process persist even during the subsequent professional life.

I have tried to bring out this practical record book so as to cover almost all the medicolegal cases/issues which the students may encounter during their professional career. The material is hypothetical case-based studies, which will give the students a practical overview and understand various scenarios that they may encounter subsequently. Each worksheet has been carefully designed to help the students get a thorough insight of the topic. However, the students should have a sound knowledge regarding the cases they are dealing with, and to finalize the report, they should come well prepared for the practicals and actively participate in them.

The teachers/faculty members in their part have to guide the students in filling up the proformas, which are self-explanatory in most aspects. The teachers may use the short case history given along with the proformas or may give a separate case scenario. If more than one exercise of the same topic needs to be done, then a photocopy of the same may be obtained.

It is hoped that this practical record book fills the vacuum for a standardized notebook, which is a need of the hour for the undergraduates. It is also hoped that this book will find a favorable response from the faculty like my textbook *Review of Forensic Medicine & Toxicology* and that they will not hesitate in recommending the same to their students.

Gautam Biswas

Acknowledgments

It is with immense gratitude that I acknowledge the mentoring role of (Late) Dr (Maj Gen) Ajit Singh during the early days of my career. I wish to recognize the influence of my teachers (Late) Dr BBL Aggarwal, Dr NK Aggarwal, Dr SK Verma, Dr KK Banerjee, Dr AK Tyagi and Dr Anil Kohli, who taught me to enquire, think and persist.

I would like to place on record my deepest gratitude to Dr Anil Kohli, Reader, Department of Forensic Medicine and Toxicology, UCMS and GTB Hospital, New Delhi, India and an exceptionally knowledgeable forensic expert for giving valuable suggestions and encouragement throughout the completion of this work.

I would like to express my heartfelt thanks to the following faculty members for providing the logistic support, Dr Tapas Kumar Bose, Professor and Head, Department of Forensic Medicine and Toxicology, Nilratan Sarkar Medical College, Kolkata, West Bengal, India; Dr Suresh K Dhattarwal, Professor and Head, Department of Forensic Medicine and Toxicology, Pt Bhagwat Dayal Sharma Postgraduate Institute of Medical Sciences, Rohtak, Haryana, India; Dr Swapnil S Agarwal, Professor and Head, Department of Forensic Medicine and Toxicology, Pramukhswami Medical College and Shree Krishna Hospital, Anand, Gujarat, India; Dr Pradeep Kumar MV, Professor, Department of Forensic Medicine and Toxicology, Rajarajeswari Medical College and Hospital, Bengaluru, Karnataka, India; Dr Sandesh Chaudhari, Associate Professor, Department of Forensic Medicine, CM Medical College, Durg, Chhattisgarh, India.

Last but not the least, I would also like to express my sincerest thanks to Mr Ravikant Rai, Area Manager, Jaypee Brothers Medical Publishers, New Delhi, who has encouraged and helped me in shaping up this record book. He is my dear friend and closely associated with my work for the last few years. I would also like to thank Mr Ramesh Kumar of our department who helped me in typing the manuscript.

Mr Prem Kumar Gupta, Secretary, Managing Society, and Professor Sandeep Puri, Principal, Dayanand Medical College and Hospital, Ludhiana, Punjab, India deserve special mention for their continuous support, inspiration and encouragement. I would also like to express my thanks to Dr Praveen Sobti, Professor, Department of Pediatrics, Christian Medical College, Ludhiana for her blessings and invaluable suggestions.

I cannot find enough words to express my gratitude to Jaypee Brothers Medical Publishers (P) Ltd, New Delhi, India for their acceptance in publishing the work, and their professionalism during the entire process. I am especially grateful to Shri Jitendar P Vij (Group Chairman), Mr Ankit Vij (Group President), Ms Chetna Vohra (Associate Director), Ms Payal Bharti (Project Manager), Mr Samir Khan (Project Coordinator), Mr Harsh Pal Singh Rawat (Graphic Designer), Mr Subhash Sarogi and Mr Pradeep Kumar (Typesetters) for shaping up the record book and making all the changes, without any complaints.

This work would not have been possible without the blessings, unconditional love, support and encouragement of my family, my parents and my in-laws throughout my life. I would like to express my love and thanks to my son, Gaurav and my earnest gratitude and love to my wife, Anupama, for her constant support and encouragement. Finally, I would like to express my sincere thanks to the Almighty for giving me the strength to complete this project.

From the Publisher's Desk
We request all the readers to provide us their valuable suggestions/errors (if any)
*at: **jppgmee@gmail.com***
so as to help us in further improvement of this book in the subsequent edition.

Contents

UNIT I: MEDICAL JURISPRUDENCE AND LEGAL PROCEDURE

UNIT II: IDENTIFICATION

UNIT III: STUDY OF MUSEUM SPECIMENS AND SLIDES

UNIT IV: MEDICOLEGAL REPORT/ INJURY REPORT

UNIT V: SEXUAL OFFENCES

UNIT VI: DEATH CERTIFICATION

UNIT VII: POSTMORTEM EXAMINATION

UNIT VIII: PROJECT

Certificate

This is certified that Mr/Ms ______________________________

of ____(College),

bearing Roll No.____________ has attended all the practicals entered in this Record Book and his/ her progress has been found satisfactory.

____

Signature of Head of the Department
(With seal)

This Practical & Postmortem Record Book has been presented for the University Practical Examination held in the year ______________.

____

Signature of the Examiner

Index

Sl. No.	Date	Exercise	Page No.	Signature of Teacher

Sl. No.	Date	Exercise	Page No.	Signature of Teacher

Sl. No.	Date	Exercise	Page No.	Signature of Teacher

Postmortem Examination Reports

Sl. No.	Date	Cause of death	Page No.	Signature of Teacher
1.				
2.				
3.				
4.				
5.				
6.				
7.				
8.				
9.				
10.				

Instructions to the Students for Practical Classes

- The students should attend all the practicals and should maintain punctuality
- They should wear a clean white lab coat with a name tag during the practicals
- They should maintain silence and discipline during all practical works. Mobile phones should be kept in the switched off mode
- They should bring the practical files during their classes and should carry one ballpen, ruler, hand lens and colored pencils
- They should listen carefully to the instructions given by the teacher for a particular practical and should come well prepared for the same. In case of any doubt, they should ask the relevant questions
- They should write the practicals accordingly, make entries in the index of the practical file and get it signed by the teacher. If a student has not finished a practical, he/she should complete it on his/her own and get the practical file checked from the concerned teacher on the next working day
- They shall be marked as absent in the subsequent class, if found to be with incomplete work
- They should avoid spillage, and cleanliness at the site of work should be maintained at all times
- Diagrams should be made by using proper color code for various structures.

General Instructions for the Examination of a Patient and Filling up of Proformas

The examination of a patient should take place in adequate light, after making the patient comfortable, maintaining privacy, in the presence of a female attendant (if a male doctor examining a female patient) and after taking informed consent for the examination and intervention.

In all the certificates issued by the medical practitioner, the names of the doctor and the patient (examinee) should be complete and in capitals (block letters) and not initials. The address should be properly written with the house number (apartment/unit number), street, nearby landmark, city/town, state, pin code and mobile number mentioned, wherever possible.

UNIT I

Medical Jurisprudence and Legal Procedure

DECLARATION

At the time of registration with the State Medical Council, each applicant is given a copy of the following declaration by the Registrar concerned, and the applicant needs to certify that he/ she has read and agree to abide by the same:

a. I solemnly pledge myself to consecrate my life to service of humanity
b. Even under threat, I will not use my medical knowledge contrary to the laws of humanity
c. I will maintain the utmost respect for human life from the time of conception
d. I will not permit considerations of religion, nationality, race, party politics or social standing to intervene between my duty and my patient
e. I will practice my profession with conscience and dignity
f. The health of my patient will be my first consideration
g. I will respect the secrets which are confined in me
h. I will give to my teachers the respect and gratitude which is their due
i. I will maintain by all means in my power, the honor and noble traditions of medical profession
j. I will treat my colleagues with all respect and dignity
k. I shall abide by the Code of Medical Ethics as enunciated in the Indian Medical Council (Professional Conduct, Etiquette and Ethics) Regulations 2002.

I make these promises solemnly, freely and upon my honor.

Place ____________________ Signature ____________________

Date ____________________ Name ____________________

Address ____________________

____

EX. 1.1: PRESCRIPTION WRITING

Write drug therapy for Amit Banerjee, 45-year-old male, residing at Quarter No 1567, Lodi Road Colony, New Delhi, who is found to be hypertensive during routine medical examination. His height is 174 cm and weight is 82 kg and BP is 160/ 118 mm Hg. No other abnormality found.

____________________________________ (Doctor's name)

______________________________ (Qualification)

______________________________ (State Medical Council Registration Number)

____ (Full Address)

__________________ (Clinic Telephone No.) ____________________________ (E-mail ID)

Prescription Serial No. ________________ Date ______________

Patient's Name ____________________________________ Age__________ Gender ____________

Contact details ____(Complete address of patient)

Mobile number __________________ E-mail ID ____________________

Diagnosis __________________________ Weight ______________
(for pediatric patients)

℞

1. ___________________________________(Generic name of medicine in capital letters only)
(Strength, dosage form, dosage instruction, duration and total quantity)

2. ____(–do–)

3. ____(–do–)

( )
Doctor's signature and date
Seal

DISPENSED
Date:_________ Name of Pharmacist:__________________

Address of Pharmacist/ Medical Store ____

EX. 1.2: BIRTH INTIMATION REPORT

Prepare a birth intimation report about Kadambari Chaurasia, 27-year-old female, wife of Shiv Kumar Chaurasia residing at House No. 324/ 25-A, Habiowal Kalan, Ludhiana, Punjab who delivered a healthy female child at Dayanand Medical College and Hospital, Ludhiana on _____________ at 12.15 AM.

Legal Information

This part to be added to birth register To be filled by the informant	
1. Date of birth	
2. Sex	
3. Name of child	
4. Name of father	
5. Name of mother	
6. Place of birth 1. Hospital/ Institution Name: Address: 2. House: 3. Other:	
7. Informant's Name: Address:	
Date: Signature or left thumb mark of the informant	

Procedure (Item number)

1. Enter the exact day, month and year the child was born, e.g. 1.1.2015
2. Enter 'male' or 'female', do not use abbreviation
3. If not named, leave blank

4&5. Full name as usually written

6. Tick the appropriate entry and give the name of the Hospital/ Institution or the address of the house where the birth took place.
8. Place where the mother usually lives.

10&11. Enter completed level of education.

12&13. If no occupation write 'Nil'.

14. If married more than once, age at first marriage.
16. Number of children born alive, to include those from earlier marriage.

To be detached and sent for statistical processing

8. **Town or village of residence of the mother:**
   a. Name of the Town/ Village
   b. Is it a town or village (*Tick '✓'*)
      ☐ Town
      ☐ Village
   c. Name of District:
   d. Name of State:
9. **Religion of the family:** (*Tick '✓'*)
   ☐ Hindu
   ☐ Muslim
   ☐ Christian
   ☐ Others (write name of the religion)
10. **Father's level of Education:**
11. **Mother's level of Education:**
12. **Father's Occupation:**
13. **Mother's Occupation:**
14. **Age of the mother at the time of marriage:** (in completed years)
15. **Age of the mother at the time of this birth:** (in completed years)
16. **Number of children born alive to the mother so far including this child:**
17. **Type of attention at delivery:** (*Tick '✓'*)
    ☐ Institutional – Government
    ☐ Institutional – Private or Non-Government
    ☐ Doctor, Nurse or Trained midwife
    ☐ Traditional Birth Attendant
    ☐ Relatives or others
18. **Method of Delivery:** (*Tick '✓'*)
    ☐ Normal
    ☐ Caesarean
    ☐ Forceps/ Vacuum
19. **Birth weight** (in kgs):
20. **Duration of pregnancy** (in weeks):

In the case of multiple births, fill in a separate form for each child and write 'Twin birth' or 'Triple birth, etc. as the case may be.

EX. 1.3: DEATH INTIMATION REPORT

Prepare a death intimation report for S. Babu Rao, 78-year-old male, son of Late Mr. GS Subramanian, residing at House No. 87-A, Anna Nagar (West), Chennai who died at KM College and Hospital, Chennai on ____________ at 7.25 PM due to renal failure of 7 days duration resulting from chronic nephritis which was diagnosed 10 years back. He was a chronic smoker for the last 50 years and was also suffering from diabetes and hypertension for 8 years.

Legal Information

This part to be added to Death Register To be filled by the informant	
1. Date of death	
2. Name of deceased	
3. Permanent address	
4. Name of father/ mother/ husband	
5. Sex of deceased	
6. Age of deceased	
7. Place of death 1. Hospital/ Institution Name: Address: 2. House: 3. Other:	
8. Informant's Name: Address:	
Date: Signature or left thumb mark of the informant	

To be detached and sent for statistical processing

9. **Town or Village of Residence of the Deceased:**
   a. Name of the Town/ Village
   b. Is it a town or village (*Tick '✓'*)
      ☐ Town
      ☐ Village
   c. Name of District:
   d. Name of State:
10. **Religion:** (*Tick '✓'*)
    ☐ Hindu
    ☐ Muslim
    ☐ Christian
    ☐ Any other religion (write name of the religion)
11. **Occupation of the Deceased:**
12. **Type of the medical attention received before death** (*Tick '✓'*):
    ☐ Institutional
    ☐ Medical attention other than institution
    ☐ No medical attention
13. **Was the cause of death medically certified** (*Tick '✓'*):
    ☐ Yes
    ☐ No
14. **Name of disease or actual cause of death**
15. **In case of this is a female death did the death occur while pregnant, at the time of delivery or within six weeks after the end of pregnancy:** (*Tick '✓'*)
    ☐ Yes
    ☐ No
16. **If use to habitually smoke for how many years?**
17. **If used to habitually chew tobacco in any form–for how many years?**
18. **If used to habitually chew arecanut in any form (including pan masala)–for how many years?**
19. **If used to habitually drink alcohol for how many years?**

EX. 1.4: STILLBIRTH INTIMATION REPORT

Meena Kumari, 23-year-old female with uncontrolled hypertension and proteinuria (diagnosed with coarctation of midabdominal aorta), delivered a stillborn baby at 29 weeks. She did not register for antenatal care (ANC). Inform the authorities regarding this.

Legal Information

To be filled by the informant (After completing all items 1 to 12, informants will put date and signature after item 6)	
1. Date of birth	
2. Sex	
3. Name of father	
4. Name of mother	
5. Place of birth: 1. Hospital/ Name: Institution 2. House Address: 3. Other place	
6. Informant's Name: Address:	
Date: Signature or left thumb mark of the informant	

To be detached and sent for statistical processing

7. **Town or Village of residence of the mother:**
   a. Name of the Town/ Village:
   b. Is it a town or village: (*Tick '✓'*)
      ☐ Town
      ☐ Village
   c. Name of District:
   d. Name of State:
8. **Age of the mother (in completed years) at the time of this birth:**
9. **Mother's level of education:**
10. **Type of attention at delivery:** (*Tick '✓'*)
    ☐ Institutional-Government
    ☐ Institutional-Private or Non-Government
    ☐ Doctor, Nurse or Trained midwife
    ☐ Traditional Birth Attendant
    ☐ Relatives or others
11. **Duration of pregnancy: (in weeks)**
12. **Cause of fetal death: (if known)**

Instructions (Item number)

1. Enter the exact day, month and year, e.g. 1–1–2015.
2. Enter 'male' or 'female', do not use abbreviation.

3&4. Full name as usually written.

5. Tick the appropriate entry below and give the name of the Hospital/ Institution or the address of the house where the birth took place, e.g. 1. Hospital.
7. Place where the mother usually lives.
9. Enter the completed level of education, e.g. if studied up to class VII but passed only class VI, write class VI.

In the case of multiple births, fill in a separate form for each child and write 'Twin birth' or 'Triple birth', etc. as the case may be.

EX. 1.5: SICKNESS CERTIFICATE

Prepare a sickness certificate for 2 weeks for Jatin Pandey, 24-year-old male, residing at Quarter No. 657/ A, Defense Colony, New Delhi, who is suffering for pneumonia which was diagnosed clinically and confirmed by laboratory tests. He has a small black mole 0.1 × 0.1 cm on the tip of his nose and a linear white scar mark measuring 1.5 × 0.5 cm on his right cheek.

Report No.__________________

Signature or thumb impression of the patient [ ]

(To be filled in by the applicant in the presence of the Government Medical Practitioner)

Identification marks:

1. ____
2. ____

I, Dr. ____ after careful examination hereby certify that

Mr/ Ms ____ S/ D/ W of _____________________________________

aged about ________ years, residing at ____ and whose

signature/ thumb impression is verified above is suffering from _____________________________________.

I consider that a period of absence from duty of ____ with effect from

____ is absolutely necessary for the restoration of his/ her health.

( )

Place ________________ Signature and Seal of Medical Practitioner

Date ________________ Registration No. ____________________

(Medical Council of India/ State Medical Council of ……….….... State)

Note: The nature and probable duration of the illness should also be specified. This certificate must be accompanied by a brief resume of the case giving the nature of the illness, its symptoms, causes and duration.

EX. 1.6: FITNESS CERTIFICATE

Draft a fitness certificate for Jatin Pandey, 24-year-old male, residing at Quarter No 657/ A, Defense Colony, New Delhi, who has recovered from pneumonia and to report on duty, for whom you issued a sickness certificate 2 weeks back. He has a small black mole 0.1 × 0.1 cm on the tip of his nose and a linear white scar mark measuring 1.5 × 0.5 cm on his right cheek.

Report No.__________________

Signature or thumb impression of the patient

(To be filled in by the applicant in the presence of the Government Medical Practitioner)

Identification marks:

1. ____
2. ____

This is to certify that I, Dr ____ have carefully examined Mr/ Ms ____________________________________ S/ W/ D of __________________________________, aged about ________________________ years, resident of _________________________________ and whose signature/ thumb impression is verified above and found that he/ she has completely recovered from his/ her illness. He/ She is now fit to resume duties in Government/ private service with effect from __________________________.

I also certify that before arriving at this decision, I have examined the original medical certificate and statement of the case on which leave was granted or extended and have taken them into consideration in arriving at my decision.

( )

Place ________________ Signature and Seal of Medical Practitioner

Date _________________ Registration No. ____________________

(Medical Council of India/ State Medical Council of …………...…. State)

Note: This certificate must be accompanied by a brief resume of the case giving the nature of the illness, its symptoms, causes and duration.

EX. 1.7: CERTIFICATE OF MEDICAL FITNESS

(To be deposited at the time of joining and obtained only from Gazetted Government Medical Practitioner)

Draft a medical fitness certificate for job recruitment for Bimal Dass, 21-year-old male, height 176 cm and weight 75 kg. He has a black mole of size 0.1 × 0.1 cm on his right side forehead just above the eyebrow and a birthmark measuring 1.5 × 1.0 cm on his left thumb on its outer aspect.

Report No.____________________

Name ____

Father's name ____

Blood group____________ Height________ cm Weight _________ kg

Chest ____

Heart and Lungs ____

Vision Left ______________________________ Right______________________________

Color vision ____

Hearing ____

Hernia/ Hydrocele/ Piles ____

Any other disease diagnosed in past ____

Allergies, if any ____

List of prescribed medication, If any:

1. ____________________________
2. ____________________________
3. ____________________________

Any other remarks: ____

I certify that I have carefully examined Mr/ Ms ____

son/ daughter of Mr ____ who has signed in my presence.

He/ she has no physical disease and is FIT.

Signature of the candidate

Place _________________

Date _________________

____

Signature of Medical Practitioner

Name, Designation and Seal

EX. 1.8A: MEDICAL EXAMINATION OF DOCK WORKERS

[For the competent person under The Dock Workers (Safety, Health and Welfare) Act 1986]

Draft a medical fitness certificate for dock worker (who loads and unloads cargo from ships onto trucks or railroad cars and verifies its contents) Atul Bhimri, 23-year-old male, height 170 cm and weight 58 kg. He has a black mole of 0.2 × 0.2 cm on left ala of his nose and a linear white scar mark measuring 1.5 × 0.5 cm on his right cheek.

Report No. ____________________

Date of Examination ________________ Date of last Examination ______________

I. Personal data

Name________________________________ Age ______________ years Gender ____________

Designation ________________________ Plant ____________ Employee Code No ____________

Identification marks: 1. ____

2. ____

II. Occupational history

1. Present occupation ____

2. Type of work being done ____

   (a) In the present occupation ____

   (b) In the previous occupation ____

3. Years of service _____________

III. Personal history

1. Smoking: Yes/ No If yes, duration ________ No. of packs per day ________________

2. Alcohol ____________________ Occasional/ Regular________________

3. Others: (Tobacco, Pan, Bhang, etc.) ____

4. Family details: Married/ Unmarried No. of children ________________

IV. Job specific personal protective equipments used (Mandatory/ Other than Mandatory)

____

V. History of past illness ___________________________________

VI. History of present illness: *Present complaints and duration* ____________________

____

VII. General Examination

Height __________ cm

Weight ____________ kg

Pulse _______ /min

BP ____________ mm Hg

Nutritional status: Normal/ Undernourished/ Malnourished/ Obese

Personal hygiene ____________________

Cyanosis: Present/ Absent

Pallor: Present/ Absent

Skin____________________

Clubbing: Present/ Absent

Edema: Present/ Absent

Any other ______________

Blood group ____________

VIII. Systemic Examination

1. Central Nervous System ______________________________
2. Cardiovascular System ______________________________
3. Respiratory System ______________________________
4. Gastrointestinal System ______________________________

   Liver ________________ Spleen ________________
5. Others ______________________________

IX. Investigations

1. Titmus Vision Test ______________________________
2. ECG ______________________________
3. Audiometry ______________________________
4. PFR ______________________________
5. Others ______________________________

____

Place ____________________

Signature of Medical Practitioner

Date ____________________

Name and Seal of the Empanelled Doctor

Registration No. and Date.........................

EX. 1.8B: FITNESS CERTIFICATE OF THE COMPETENT PERSON

[Under Dock Workers (Safety, Health and Welfare) Act 1986]

I hereby certify that I have personally examined Mr/ Ms ______________________

S/ D/ W of ______________________ residing at ______________________

who is desirous of being employed in ______________ in the capacity of ______________

and that his/ her age as nearly as can be ascertained from my examination is __________ years and that he/ she is

free from any disease or disability likely to endanger him and others on employment in ______________

in the capacity of ______________ and hence I declare him physically and mentally fit for employment.

Reason for:

i. Refusal of fitness certificate ______________________

ii. Certificate being revoked ______________________

______________________ ______________________

Signature/ Left thumb impression of the person

Signature of Medical Practitioner
Name and Seal of the Empanelled Doctor

Place ______________

Registration No. and Date ______________

Date ______________

Note:

1. Certificate to be supported by the results of medical examination and investigation results in the prescribed proforma.
2. Exact details of the cause of physical disability should be clearly stated.
3. Functional/ Productive abilities should be stated, if disability is stated.

EX. 1.9: CERTIFICATE OF EXAMINATION OF AN ARRESTED PERSON

Draft a certificate for Sayed Hussain, 40-year-old male, residing at 456/ 35-C, Mohalla Shiv Puri, Janakpuri, New Delhi who was arrested by the police for alleged murder of his business partner and brought for examination. He has a black mole of 0.2 × 0.1 cm on his right ear and a linear white scar mark measuring 8.5 × 2.5 cm on his left forearm on its outer aspect.

Report No. ________________ Date ____________

As per requisition from ______________________________ dated ____________________, physical examination of

Mr/ Ms ______________________________________ S/ D/ W of ____,

residing at ____, involved in FIR No. ____________________

of police station ___________________________ was done on _________________ at _______________ AM/ PM.

Consent	**Identification marks**
I have voluntary agreed for the medical examination and investigations. I have been explained that it was necessary for diagnosis and treatment of the disease from which I may be suffering. This has been explained in _________________ language which I understand. Signature/ Thumb impression of the examinee	1. ______________________________ ______________________________ 2. ______________________________ ______________________________

History (related to illness/ injury, if any) ____

Physical Examination

A. General: Build and nourishment: Poor/ Moderate/ Obese

Height _______ cm   Weight _______ kg.   Pulse _______ /min

Blood pressure_________ mm Hg   Pallor: Present/ Absent

Physical deformity, if any ____

Others, if any: ____

B. Systemic Examination

1. Central Nervous System ____
2. Cardiovascular System ____
3. Respiratory System ____
4. Gastrointestinal System ____

C. Injuries, if any (use body diagrams) ____

D. Investigations, if any ____

Opinion

There is no evidence of any clinically identifiable illness.

There are no injuries on the person/ injuries on the person which could be caused as alleged.*

Suggestions, if any ____

Place ___________ Signature of Medical Practitioner

Date___________ Name, Designation and Seal

*(strike off which is not applicable)

EX. 1.10: HEALTH SCREENING OF PRISONERS ON ADMISSION TO JAIL

Draft a certificate for Joseph Mathew, 40-year-old male, residing at 95/ A, Gali No. 2, Andheri (East) Mumbai who was sentenced to 5 years prison for armed robbery. He has a black mole of 0.5 × 0.5 cm on this right side forehead and a hairy elevated mole of 1× 1 cm on his chin.

Report No. ______________ Date ______________

Name ______________________________ Age ______ years Gender ______________

Father's/ Husband's name ______________________________ Occupation ______________

Date and time of admission in the prison ______________________________

Consent	Identification marks
I have voluntary agreed for the medical examination and investigations. I have been explained that it was necessary for diagnosis and treatment of the disease from which I may be suffering. This has been explained in ______________ language which I understand. Signature/ Thumb impression of the examinee	1. ______________ ______________ 2. ______________ ______________

Previous History of illness

Are you suffering from any disease(s)? Yes/ No

If so, the name of the disease(s) ______________________________

Are you now taking medicines for the same? ______________________________

Are you suffering from cough that has lasted for 3 weeks or more Yes/ No

History of drug abuse, if any ______________________________

Any information the prisoner may volunteer ______________________________

Physical Examination

Height ________ cm Weight ________ kg Last menstruation period ______________

1. Pallor: Yes/ No
2. Lymph node enlargement: Yes/ No
3. Clubbing: Yes/ No
4. Cyanosis: Yes/ No
5. Icterus: Yes/ No
6. Injury, if any:

Any other ______________________________

Systemic Examination

1. Central Nervous System ____________________
2. Cardiovascular System ____________________
3. Respiratory System ____________________
4. Eye, ENT ____________________
5. Gastrointestinal System ____________________
6. Teeth and Gums ____________________
7. Urinary System ____________________

Sample taken: Blood for Hepatitis/ STD including HIV (with the informed consent of the prisoner whenever required by law)

Date of completion of medical investigation ____________________

Opinion

There is no evidence of identifiable illness.

There is evidence of ____________________ illness.

Suggestions/ Advice given ____________________

____

Place ____________ Signature of Medical Practitioner

Date ____________ Name, Designation and Seal

EX. 1.11: CONSENT TO SURGERY, DIAGNOSTIC PROCEDURES OR OTHER MEDICAL PROCEDURES

Sheela Devi (gravida 5, para 5), a 65-year-old female, weighing 50 kg, having third degree uterovaginal prolapse for 10 years is admitted with complaints of vaginal bleeding and severe pelvic pain for 3 months. She is posted for vaginal hysterectomy and pelvic floor repair. Take an informed consent for the same explaining the procedure that you are going to follow, anesthesia to be administered (local, regional or general), other alternatives, and important complications (hemorrhage, infections, embolism, damage to adjacent organs and adverse reaction to anesthesia).

Patient's particulars

Patient's name ______________________________

Age ______________ Gender ______________

Procedure is explained

I approve and direct Dr.(s) ______________________________ or other doctors judged qualified by him or her to perform a ______________________________

Types of medicines given

Sedation and Anesthesia

This procedure will be done with: *(Tick '✓')*

☐ No sedation (medicines used to make you calm, drowsy, or fall asleep)
☐ Small amount of sedation
☐ Moderate or conscious sedation
☐ Deep sedation
☐ Anesthesia (pain medicine that will keep you from feeling anything).

Risks are explained

The risks, benefits, alternatives and complications of sedation have been explained and my questions answered. I, the patient, or someone representing me, has approved the plan for sedation.

My doctor may need to do other procedures during this surgery or procedure. This could happen if he or she finds an unexpected condition. If my doctor feels it's needed, I agree to these added procedures. These would be done to avoid the risks of having a second surgery or procedure.

I understand the purpose of the surgery or procedure needed for my treatment. I know the practice of medicine, surgery, and dentistry is not an exact science. I know that no guarantee can be made about the outcome.

Questions so far?

Do you have a question? Please ask or write your question below.

____

Signature of patient ______________

Risk are explained

Risks

I understand the medical risks and results including:

____

I also understand there are general risks with surgery or invasive procedures. These risks are: infection, bleeding, injury to surrounding structures, stroke, paralysis and death.

These risks have been explained to me.

Benefits are explained

Benefits

I also know the benefits including ______________________________

Other options are given here

Other Options

I have been told of any reasonable other treatment choices. I know the risks and results of these other choices. These include, but are not limited to:

____

I have also been told of the risks and results of having no treatment:

____

Consent begins here

Consent for Use of Tissue, Organs and Body Parts

Unless I say otherwise, I allow ______________________ to save and use any tissue, organs or other body parts removed during the surgery or other procedures. They may dispose of these by standard medical practice. I give up any claim I may have to this tissue, organ or other body part once removed.

Consent to Take Part in Medical Research, Study or Education Related

I agree to have pictures taken for medical study or research. I agree to the first copying or publication of these pictures, as long as my identity is kept secret. Is a teaching hospital, to advance medical education, I also agree to allow observers, technical representatives and participants in the operating room. I also understand that I may have a physical examination for educational reasons.

Questions so far?

Do you have a question? Please ask or write your question below.

____

Signature of patient ______________

More consent

Consent for Administration of Blood and Blood Products

I understand that I might need blood or blood products during the surgery, procedure, or other treatments. I may also need it in the period of time after surgery. This period is not usually longer than a week. I know there are certain risks to receiving blood and blood products.

These risks include blood reaction with fever, chills, and breathing problems, and blood-transmitted disease that may not be found by testing blood before it is given.

There may be other risks. I understand the risks of accepting blood and blood products. I consent to receive blood or blood products as believed needed in my doctor's opinion.

Understanding the process

Before you sign....let's make sure you understand everything

To make sure we have explained this well, please answer these questions:

a. The procedure I am having is called a ____________________

b. Sedation or anesthesia might be used. Sedation is ____________________, drowsy or ____________________.

c. I know there are always ____________________ to general surgery and other procedures. One of these is ____________________.

d. Along with risks, there are also ____________________ to this procedure. These are ____________________.

e. I am agreeing to have my____________________ taken for medical research or study.

Ready to sign consent form

Signatures

My signature below means that I have read and understood this consent form. I have been given all the information I asked for about the procedure(s), risks and other options. All my questions were answered. I agree to everything explained above.

Patient's signature

Patient's signature ____________________ Date ____________________

Doctor's signature

Doctor's signature ____________________ Date ____________________

Independent witness signature

Witness signature ____________________ Date ____________________

In case of minor/ insane

If the patient is not able to consent for herself, complete the following:

Patient ____________________ is not able to consent because:

____

Legally responsible person ____________________

Relationship to patient ____________________ Date signed ____________________

EX. 1.12: CONSENT FOR STERILIZATION

Sugata Pachauri w/ o of Anindya Pauchari's, a 25-year-old female (gravida 3, para 3) had her third uneventful vaginal delivery today. She is scheduled for tubal sterilization by modified Pomeroy technique tomorrow. Take informed consent from her and her husband for the same.

Date and time ___________________

We, the undersigned, Mr ____ aged _______ years, husband of Ms ____ aged _____________ years residing at ____ having _________ children (__________ male, aged ____________ years; _____________ female, aged _____________ years), of sound mind, consent for operation of ____ (state nature and extent of the operation) to be performed upon Mr/ Ms ____ by Dr(s) ____ under _____________________________ anesthesia to be administered by Dr ____ (name of the anesthetist).

We have been explained and have understood the technique of operation, the procedure of anesthesia, the consequences of operation (operation intended to result in sterility although the result has not been guaranteed; and that a sterile person is NOT capable of becoming a parent) and the risks and complications of operation and anesthesia including the remote possibility of failure of operation resulting in future pregnancy.

We understand that the procedure other than proposed ones or in addition to them, for the operation/ anesthesia may be found necessary and I consent for them, if the surgeon/ anesthetist think them essential (life saving) for the patient.

We voluntarily request the operation and understand that if it proves successful, the results will be permanent and it will thereafter be physically impossible for the patient to inseminate/ conceive to bear children.

Signatures: ________________________ ________________________

(Husband) (Wife)

Signature, Name and Registration Number of Medical Practitioner ______________________________

____

Signature of the witness ____

Name and address of witness ____

EX. 1.13A: CONSENT FOR MEDICAL TERMINATION OF PREGNANCY

Gitaben, a 31-year-old woman and her husband Padmesh Keshavlal, a street hawker presented to the family planning clinic with complaints of amenorrhea, nausea and pain in back. Ultrasound was done, and it reported pregnancy with gestational age of 16 weeks and 3 days. She wants a MTP for her fourth unplanned pregnancy as they cannot afford to rear another child. Discuss with the patient the methods that you are going to use, side effects, complications and alternative options. Take consent after the counseling session.

I, ______________________________ D/ W of ______________________________

aged ________ years, residing at ______________________________ do hereby give my consent to termination of my pregnancy at ______________________________ (place where pregnancy is to be terminated).

Place ______________ Signature ______________________

Date ______________

(To be filled by the guardian where the woman is a mentally ill person or minor)

I ______________________________ S/ D/ W of ______________________________

aged ____________ years, and residing at ______________________________ hereby give my consent to the termination of the pregnancy of my ward ______________________________ who is a minor/ of unsound mind at ______________________________ (place of termination of pregnancy).

Place ______________ Signature ______________________

Date ______________

EX. 1.13B: DETAILED CONSENT FOR MEDICAL TERMINATION OF PREGNANCY

I, the undersigned, Ms ______________________________ aged __________ years,

W/ D of ______________________________ residing at ______________________________

______________________________ admitted under CR No. ____________ with OPD No. ________

permit Dr(s) ______________________________ to terminate my pregnancy as:

☐ The pregnancy has occurred as a result of failure of the contraceptive technique of ______________ ______________ (IUD/ oral pills/ condom/ coitus interruptus/ tubectomy/ vasectomy, etc.) employed by us.

☐ This pregnancy has resulted from occurrence of unconsented forceful sexual intercourse.

☐ There is substantial risk that if the child is born, it would suffer from such physical or mental abnormalities as to be seriously handicapped

☐ The pregnancy poses risk of injury to my physical or mental health by reason of my actual/ reasonably foreseen environment.

(Tick '√' whichever is applicable)

- The procedure/s proposed to be employed for termination of pregnancy and of anesthesia have been explained to me, and I have understood the same.
- The risks and possible complications of anesthesia and operation, including the remote possibility of pregnancy continuing in spite of the MTP procedure, have been explained to me.
- I also understand that procedures other than the proposed ones, or in addition to them for termination of pregnancy, and/ or anesthetizing, may be found necessary or desirable, and I consent to them, if the surgeon and/ or the anesthetist think them essential for me.

______________________ ______________________

Signature of the witness Signature of the patient

Place ______________________

Date with time ______________________

Signature, Name and Registration Number of Medical Practitioner ______________________________

____

EX. 1.14: CONSENT FOR PRENATAL DIAGNOSTIC PROCEDURES

Mitali Vashist w/ o Kishan Vashist, a 36-year-old woman, gravida 3, para 2, came for prenatal diagnosis and treatment clinic because of the diagnoses of gestational diabetes mellitus and polyhydramnios, and abnormal results of an ultrasound examination performed by her obstetrician. Her first baby had died within 3 hours of birth; the appearance of the baby had suggested dwarfism. Her second pregnancy had been complicated by polyhydramnios, preeclampsia and gestational diabetes mellitus that ended in the birth of a stillborn male baby. Take informed consent for the procedure.

I, ____ W/D of ________________________

of age ____________ years residing at ____

hereby state that I have been explained fully the probable side effects and after effects of the prenatal diagnostic procedures. I wish to undergo the prenatal diagnostic procedures in my interest to find out the possibility of any abnormality (i.e. disease or disorder) in the child I am carrying.

I undertake not to terminate the pregnancy if the prenatal diagnostic procedure and any prenatal tests conducted show absence of deformity or disorder. I understand that the sex of the fetus will not be disclosed to me.

I understand that breach of this undertaking will make me liable to penalty as prescribed in the Prenatal Diagnostic Techniques (Regulation and Prevention of Misuse) Rules, 1994.

Place ________________ Signature ________________

Date ________________

I have explained the contents of the above consent to the patient and her companion.

(Name ____________________ Address ______________________________________

relationship ______________________________________) in the language she/ they understand.

Date ____________

Signature, Name and Registration Number of Medical Practitioner ________________________

____

Name, Address and Registration Number of the Genetic Clinic ________________________

Note: A copy of the consent is given to the patient.

EX. 1.15: INFORMATION TO HEALTH AUTHORITIES REGARDING NOTIFIABLE DISEASES

Tularam Gaitonde, a 65-year-old man is admitted in your hospital with the symptoms of H1N1 (high fever, cough, running nose etc). You had already collected the nasal swab samples and had sent them for testing, the reports of which has come to be positive. He has been kept in an isolated ward. Inform your local health authorizes regarding the same.

CASE DEFINITION ____________________

Clinical Information

Physician Name - Last Name	First Name	Telephone Number

Patient Information

Last Name	First Name	Middle Name

Father's/ Guardian's name ____________________

Age______ years Gender ☐ Male ☐ Female ☐ Other______

Pregnant ☐ Yes ☐ No ☐ Unknown If Yes, Est. Delivery Date (____/ ____/ ______)

Address ____________________

County of residence ____________ Country of birth, if not Indian born ____________

Date of arrival in India (mm/ dd/ yyyy) ____________

Telephone number __________ Mobile number ☐☐☐☐☐☐☐☐☐☐

E-mail ____________

Occupation (Describe/ Specify) ____________________

Primary Language ____________

Race (*Tick '✓'*)

☐ Indian ☐ White ☐ African-American/ Black ☐ American Indian

☐ Japanese ☐ Korean ☐ Chinese ☐ Other: ________

Signs and Symptoms

Symptomatic? ☐ Yes ☐ No ☐ Unknown	*Onset Date (mm/ dd/ yyyy)*	*Date First Sought Medical Care (mm/ dd/ yyyy)*

Signs/ Symptoms (Specify) ____________________

____

____

____

Past Medical History ______________________________

Hospitalization

Did patient visit emergency room for illness? ☐ Yes ☐ No ☐ Unknown	*Was patient hospitalized?* ☐ Yes ☐ No ☐ Unknown	*If Yes, how many total hospital nights?*

Hospitalization – Details ______________________________

Outcome

Outcome? ☐ Survived ☐ Died ☐ Unknown	*If Survived,* Survived as of ____________ *(mm/ dd/ yyyy)*	*Date of Death (mm/ dd/ yyyy)*

Laboratory Information

Specimen Type 1	*Type of Test*	*Specimen Type 2*	*Type of Test*
☐ Serum ☐ CSF ☐ Other ____________		☐ Serum ☐ CSF ☐ Other ____________	

Laboratory Results Summary – Other ______________________________

Epidemiologic Information

Travel history

Did patient travel ***outside of county of residence*** *during the incubation period?* ☐ Yes ☐ No ☐ Unknown	*Has the patient traveled outside India during the incubation period?* ☐ Yes ☐ No ☐ Unknown

If yes for either of these questions, specify all locations and dates below.

Travel history - details

Location (city, county, state, country)	Date travel started (mm/ dd/ yyyy)	Date travel ended (mm/ dd/ yyyy)

Exposures/ Risk Factors ______________________________

Reporting Agency

Investigator Name	*Local Health Jurisdiction*	*Telephone Number*	*Date (mm/ dd/ yyyy)*

First Reported By

☐ Clinician ☐ Laboratory ☐ Other (specify): ____________

State Use Only

Case Classification
☐ Confirmed ☐ Probable ☐ Suspected ☐ Not a case ☐ Need additional information

EX. 1.16: RECORDING OF DYING DECLARATION BY A MEDICAL PRACTITIONER

Chandanika Swain, a 25-year-old female, married last year, is admitted in your hospital with alleged history of being burnt by her parents-in-law and her husband who sprinkled kerosene oil on the clothes and set her on fire, and bolted the door of her room from outside. The neighbors on hearing her screaming and shouting, rescued her and brought to the hospital in critical condition. She has 95% burns. Record her dying declaration since there is no time to call the Magistrate. (Note: Take the declaration from the patient only. Do not make any cutting/ overwriting or change the pen. Do not take thumb impression in case of a 100% burn case).

I, Dr ____________________ S/ D/ W of ____________________, working as ____________________, residing at ____________________ in presence of witnesses (1) ____________________ S/ D/ W of ____________________ residing at ____________________ and witness (2) ____________________ S/ D/ W of ____________________ residing at ____________________ shall record the dying declaration of Mr/ Ms ____________________ aged about __________ years, S/ D/ W of ____________________ married/ unmarried, occupation ____________________ residing at ____________________ at __________ AM/ PM, on __________ (date), at ____________________ (place) in the word by word order as narrated by the declarant.

Certification of Compos Mentis

Questions that may be asked:

a. What is your name?
b. What is the year/ season/ date/ month?
c. Whether it is morning/ evening/ night?
d. Where do you live?
e. Where do you think you are?
f. Are you married? What is the name of your eldest sibling?
g. What is you education?

I have thoroughly examined his/ her level of consciousness, orientation of time and space, memory and other mental faculties and I hereby certify that the declarant is in possession of a sound mind to deliver his dying declaration.

I, Dr.____________________, have come to record your dying declaration.

Will you be able to answer my questions? Yes/ No

Dying Declaration

Before recording this dying declaration, I have examined the declarant and found that his/ her condition is critical and he/ she may die any time hereafter, in spite of the lifesaving treatment being given to him/ her. The words of the declarant as said by him/ her are: ______________________

In order to clarify the points as revealed by above and in continuation to this, I asked the following questions to which the declarant gave the answers, which are recorded in that sequence:

i. Why were you brought to the hospital? (describe the incident in detail since beginning)

ii. At what time the incident took place?

iii. How, by whom, under what circumstances and at which place, did you sustain injury?

iv. What is the reason behind this incident?

v. Did you have any past enemy?

vi. Who were present at the time of the incident?

vii. Anything else that you want to mention about the incident?

____

____

viii. Can you sign/ put thumb impression?

____

The above recorded dying declaration is correct as per my dictation which I am signing after reading that bear my signature/ thumb impression (should be translated into declarant's mother tongue by a translator).

I, Dr ______________________ certify that the above declaration was recorded by me.

I also certify that the declarant Mr/ Ms ______________________ maintained

his/ her sound state of mind throughout the dictation of his/ her declaration. The recording ended at ________ AM/ PM on ____________.

____

Signature of Medical Practitioner
(Name, Designation and Seal)

Signature/ Thumb impression of declarant

Place ________

Date ________

Signature of the translator ______________________

Name and address ______________________

Recorded and signed in our presence

1. Signature, Name and Address of first witness ______________________
2. Signature, Name and Address of second witness ______________________

NOTES

NOTES

NOTES

UNIT II

Identification

EX. 2.1: ESTABLISHMENT OF PERSONAL IDENTITY

A. Name: ______________________________

B. Father's/ Husband's Name: ______________________________

C. Gender: ______________________________

D. Age__________ years

E. Residential Address ______________________________

F. Identification Marks

1. ______________________________

2. ______________________________

G. Documentary Proof (Birth certificate/ Voter's card/ Passport/ Aadhar Card/ Driving License, etc.)

____

H. Thumb Impression (right thumb for females and left thumb for males)

I. Attested Photograph

EX. 2.2: ESTABLISHMENT OF IDENTITY

1. **Race and religion**
   a. Clothing ______________________
   b. Complexion ______________________
   c. Eyes ______________________
   d. Hair ______________________
   e. Teeth ______________________
   f. Feet ______________________
   g. Tattoo marks ______________________

2. **Determination of Race from:**

   Skull

   a. Cephalic Index ______________________

Type of skull	Cephalic index	Race

   b. *Other Indices*
      i. Brachial Index ______________________
      ii. Crural Index ______________________
      iii. Intermembral Index ______________________
      iv. Humerofemoral Index ______________________
      v. Nasal Index ______________________

EX. 2.3: DETERMINATION OF SEX IN LIVING (Clinical Examination)

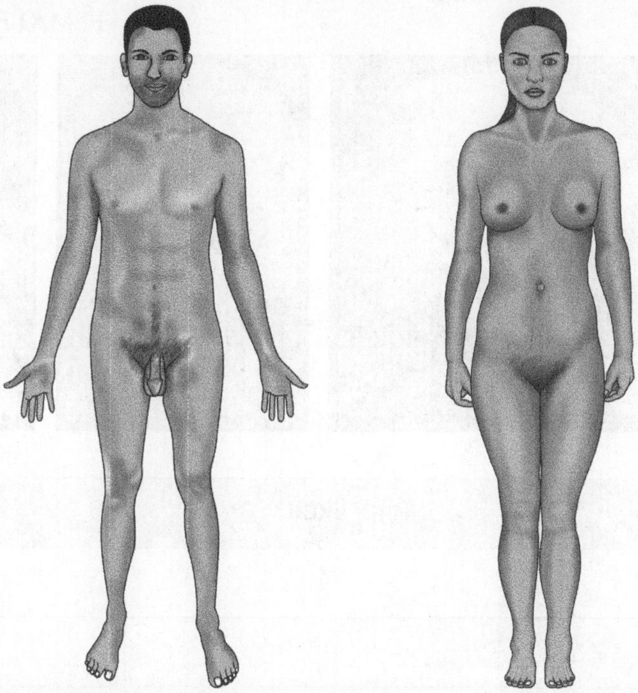

Sl. No.	Feature	Male	Female

EX. 2.4: DETERMINATION OF SEX FROM SKELETAL REMAINS (Skull)

MALE

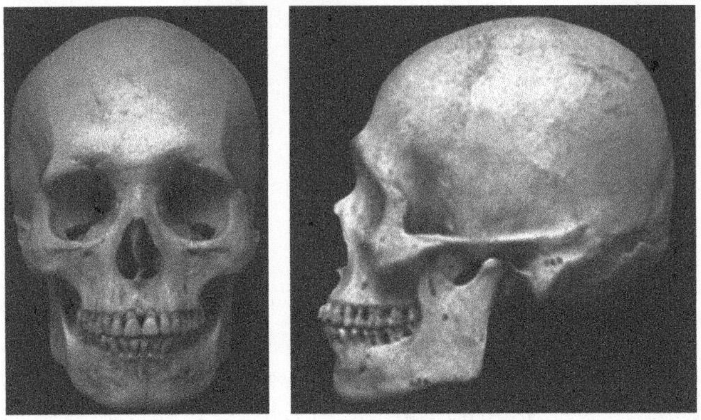

FEMALE

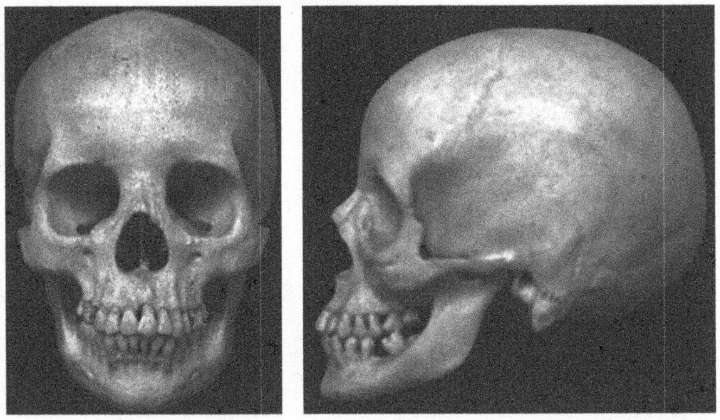

Sl. No.	Feature	Male skull	Female skull

EX. 2.5: DETERMINATION OF SEX FROM SKELETAL REMAINS (Mandible)

MALE

FEMALE

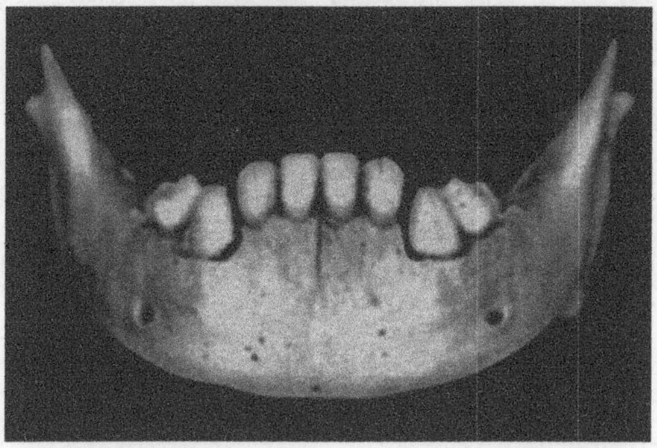

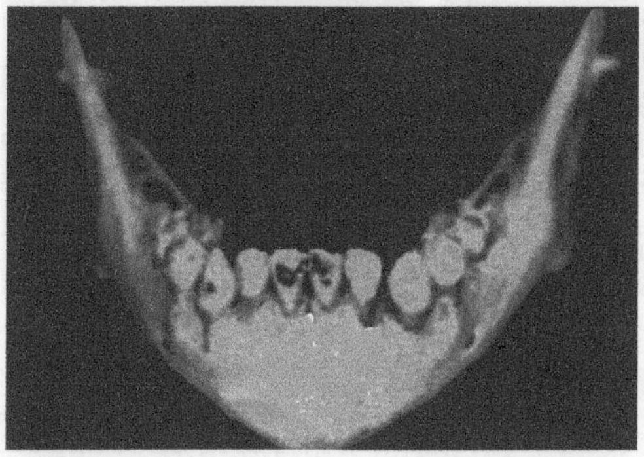

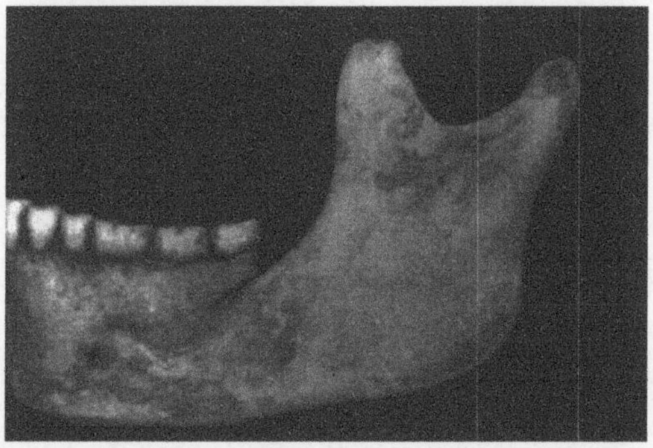

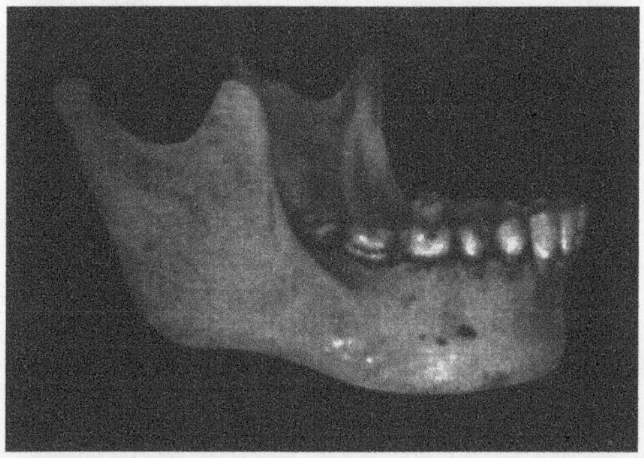

Sl. No.	Feature	Male mandible	Female mandible

EX. 2.6: DETERMINATION OF SEX FROM SKELETAL REMAINS (Pelvis)

MALE

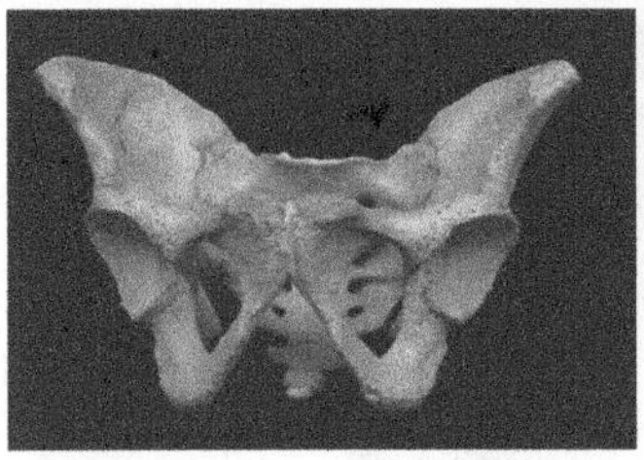

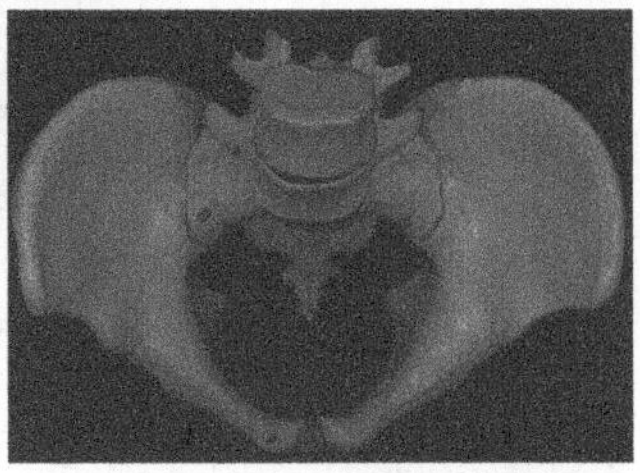

FEMALE

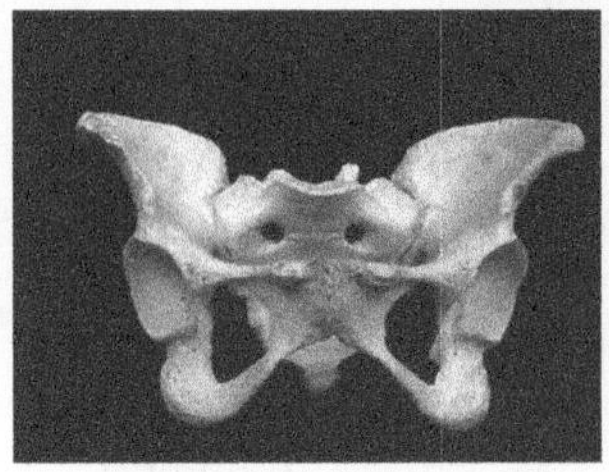

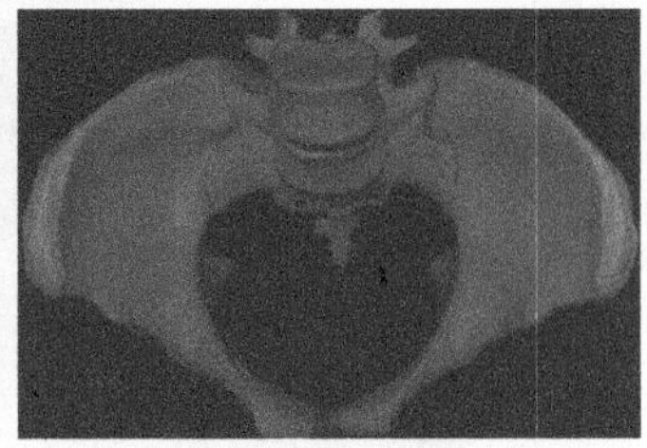

Sl. No.	Feature	Male pelvis	Female pelvis

EX. 2.7: DETERMINATION OF SEX FROM SKELETAL REMAINS (Sacrum)

MALE

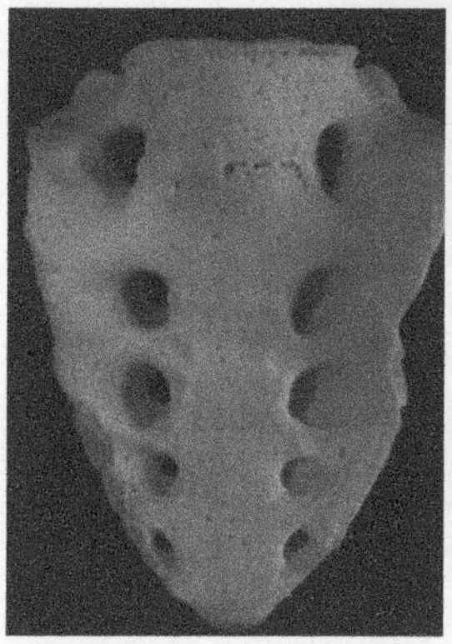

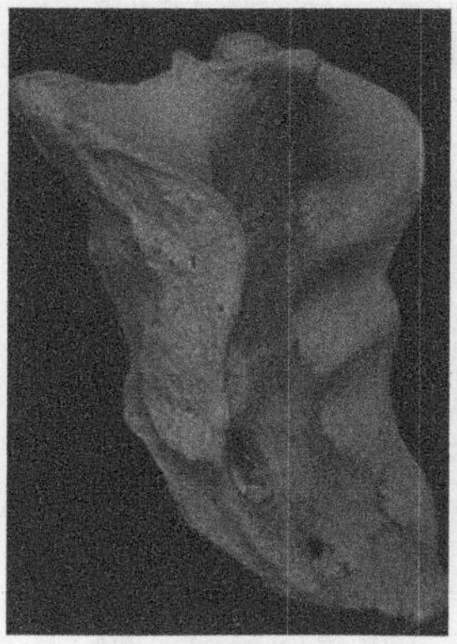

FEMALE

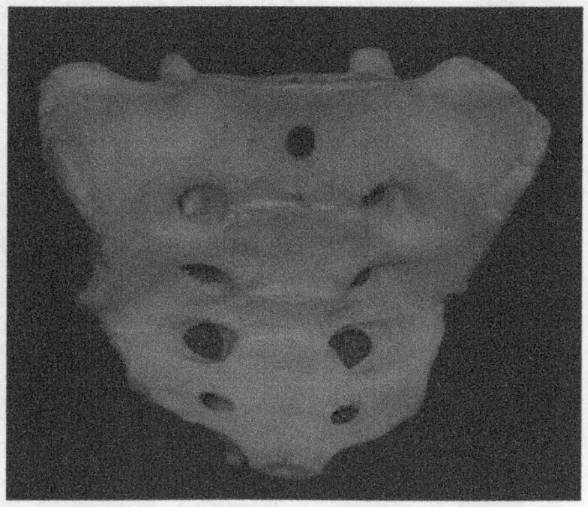

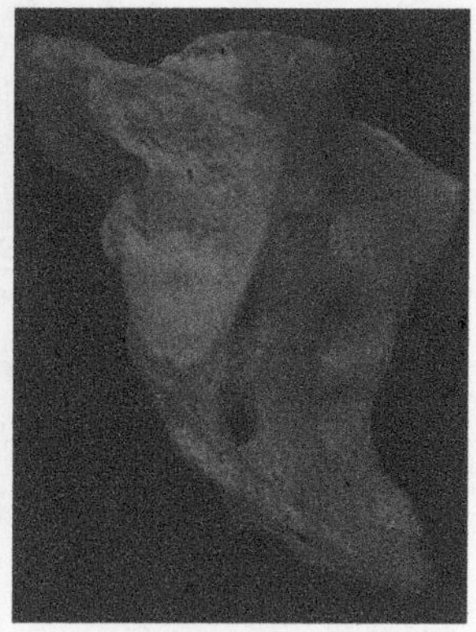

Sl. No.	Feature	Male sacrum	Female sacrum

EX. 2.8: DETERMINATION OF SEX FROM SKELETAL REMAINS (Femur)

MALE FEMALE

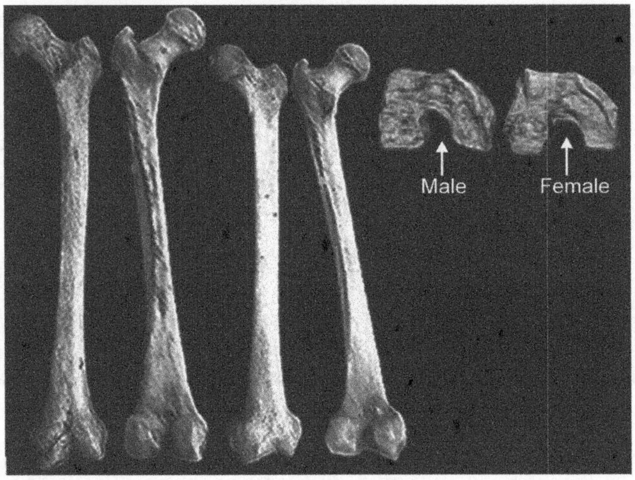

Sl. No.	Feature	Male femur	Female femur

EX. 2.9: DETERMINATION OF SEX FROM SKELETAL REMAINS (Sternum)

Sl. No.	Feature	Male sternum	Female sternum

EX. 2.10: DETERMINATION OF SEX FROM SKELETAL REMAINS (Humerus)

Sl. No.	Feature	Male humerus	Female humerus

EX. 2.11: DENTAL STUDY

A. **Teeth formation and composition** ______

B. **Temporary Teeth** ______

C. **Permanent Teeth** ______

i. *Superadded Permanent Teeth* ______

ii. *Successional Permanent Teeth* ______

D. **Spacing of Jaw** ______

E. **Period of Mixed Dentition** ______

F. **International System of Numbering of Teeth (FDI or ISO system)**

i. Permanent teeth

ii. Temporary teeth

EX. 2.12: ESTIMATION OF AGE FROM ERUPTION OF TEETH

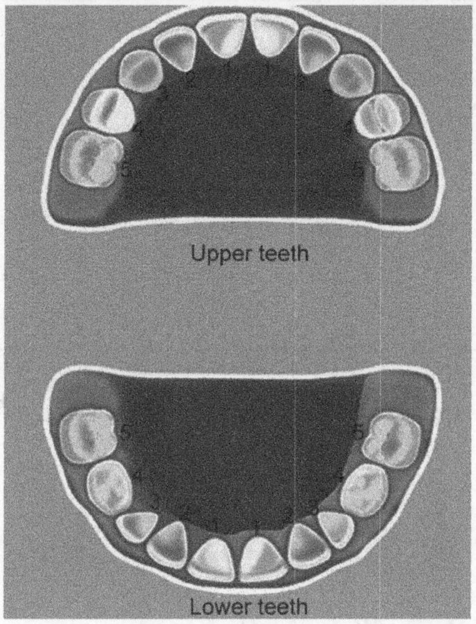

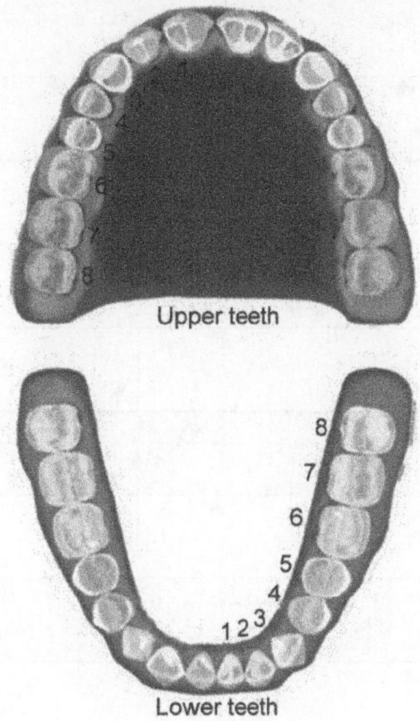

Eruption of Temporary Teeth

Teeth	Age of eruption
Central incisors Lower Upper	
Lateral incisors Upper Lower	
First molars	
Canines	
Second molars	

Eruption of Permanent Teeth

Teeth	Age of eruption
First molars	
Central incisors	
Lateral incisors	
First premolars	
Second premolars	
Canines	
Second molars	
Third molars	

Differences between Temporary and Permanent Teeth

Feature	Temporary teeth	Permanent teeth

Estimation of Age from Teeth in Elderly Subjects

a. Miles' Method ______________________________

____

b. Gustafson's Method ______________________________

Sl. No.	Criteria/ Changes	Features/ Findings

EX. 2.13: STUDY OF MANDIBLES IN DIFFERENT AGE GROUPS

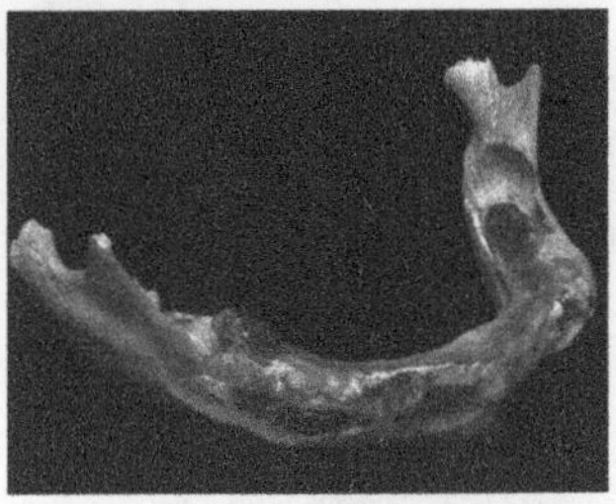

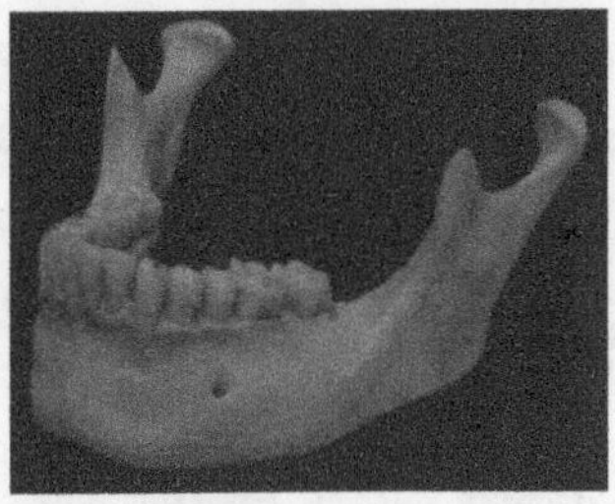

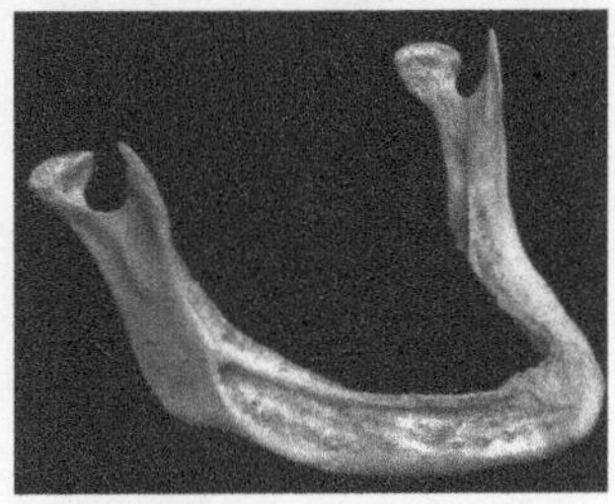

Infancy

Adult

Old age

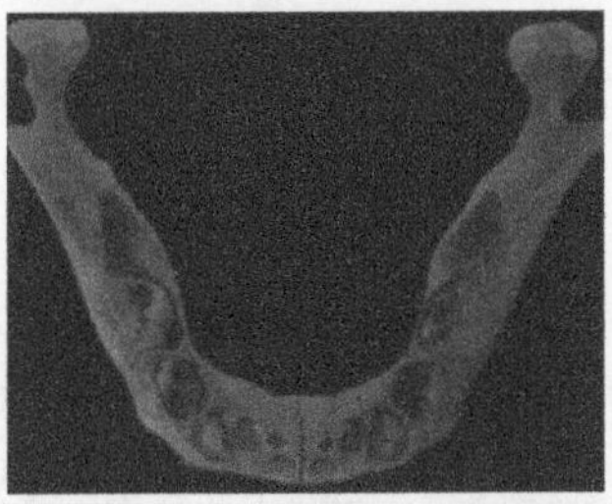

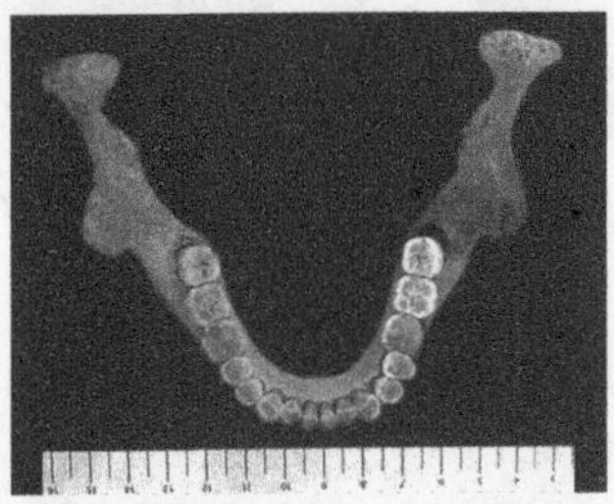

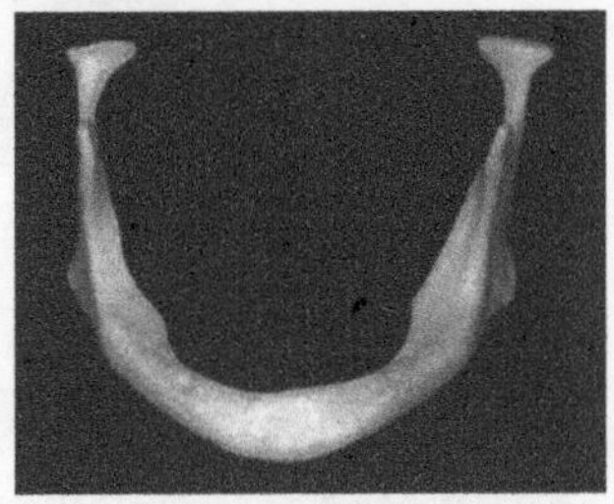

Feature	Infancy	Adult	Old age

EX. 2.14: ESTIMATION OF AGE FROM SKULL SUTURE CLOSURE

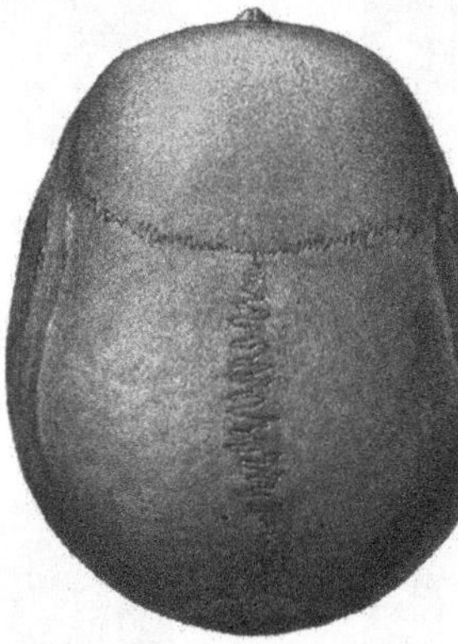

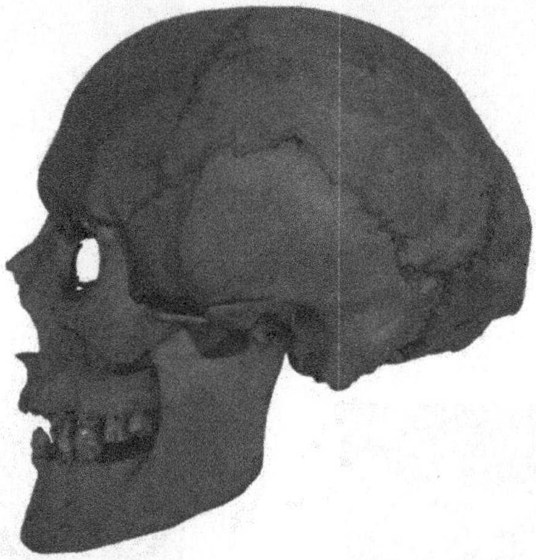

Sl. No.	Suture	Closure Age

EX. 2.15: ESTIMATION OF AGE FROM PUBIC SYMPHYSEAL SURFACE

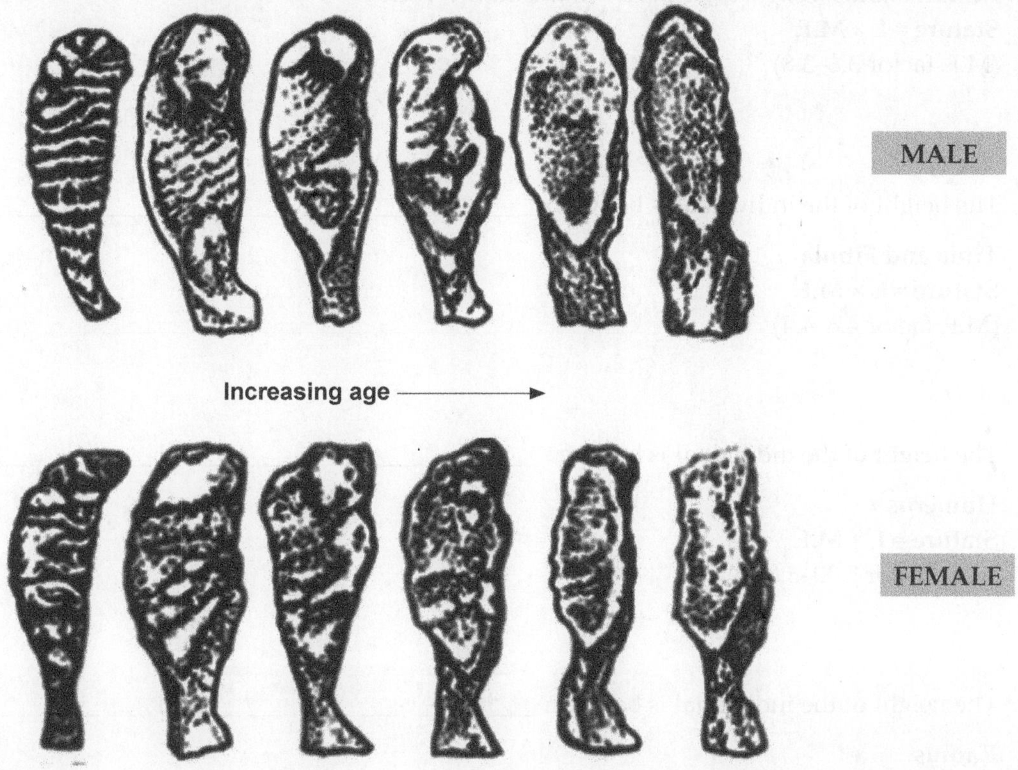

Age	Features
Below 20 years	
Between 20 and 25 years	
Between 25 and 30 years	
Between 35 and 45 years	
Between 45 and 50 years	
Above 50 years	
Above 60 years	

EX. 2.16: ESTIMATION OF STATURE FROM LONG BONES

A. **Femur:** *Stature: Length of the Bone × Multiplication Factor*
Stature = L × M.F.
(M.F. factor 3.6–3.8)

The height of the individual is between ____________ and ____________ cm.

B. **Tibia and Fibula**
Stature = L × M.F.
(M.F. factor 4.8–4.4)

The height of the individual is between ____________ and ____________ cm.

C. **Humerus**
Stature = L × M.F.
(M.F. factor 5.30–5.0)

The height of the individual is between ____________ and ____________ cm.

D. **Radius**
Stature = L × M.F.
(M.F. factor 6.7–6.9)

The height of the individual is between ____________ and ____________ cm.

E. **Ulna**
Stature = L × M.F.
(M.F. factor 6.0–6.3)

The height of the individual is between ____________ and ____________ cm.

F. **Clavicle**
Stature = L × M.F.
(M.F. factor 11.1)

The height of the individual is about ________________________ cm.

EX. 2.17: STUDY OF APPEARANCE AND FUSION OF EPIPHYSES IN YOUNG, AND SUTURE CLOSURE FOR OLD AGE

Age	Appearance of Ossification Centers	Fusion of Epiphyses
At birth		
6–7 years		
12 years		
14 years		

Age	Appearance of Ossification Centers	Fusion of Epiphyses
16 years		
18 years		
21 years		
45 years and above		

EX. 2.18A: DETERMINATION OF AGE FROM X-RAYS

Determine the age of the male individuals from the given X-rays.

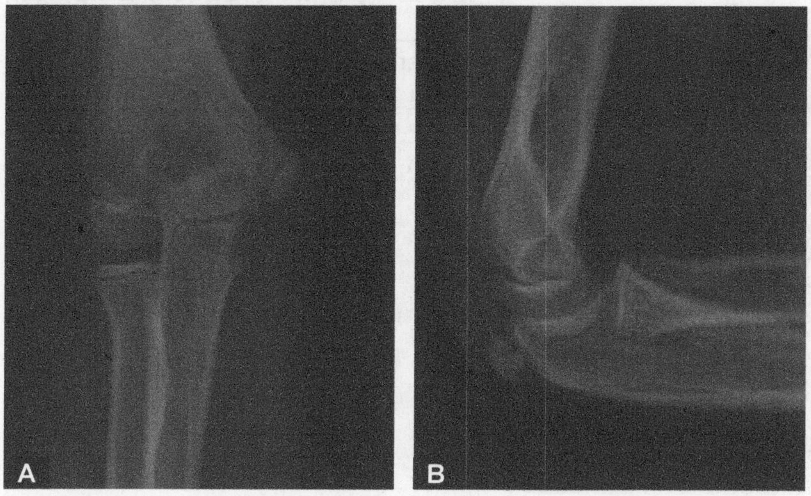

View:

Observations:

Inference:

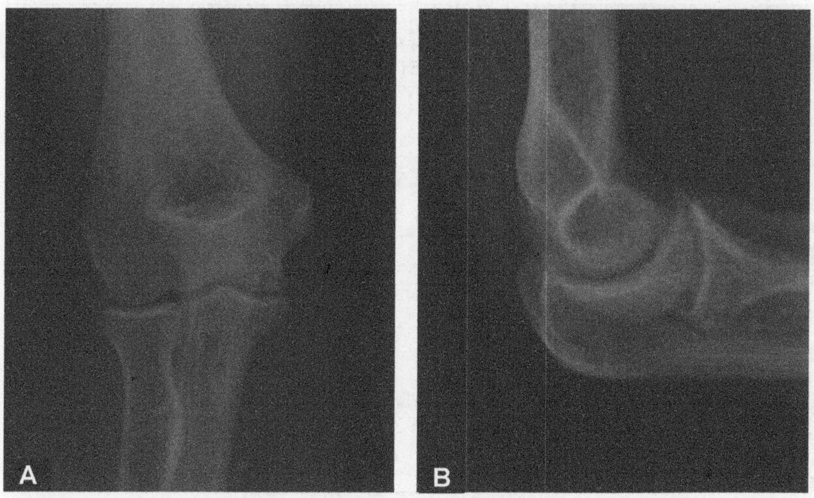

View:

Observations:

Inference:

EX. 2.18B: DETERMINATION OF AGE FROM X-RAYS

Determine the age of the male individuals from the given X-rays.

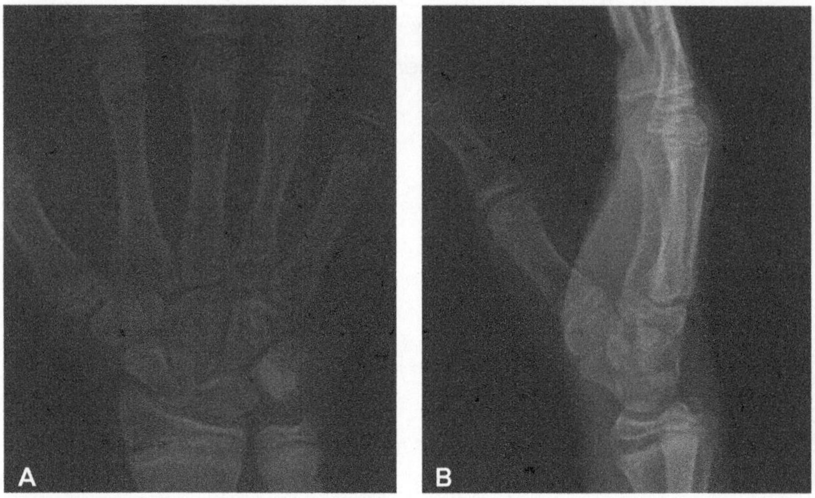

View:

Observations:

Inference:

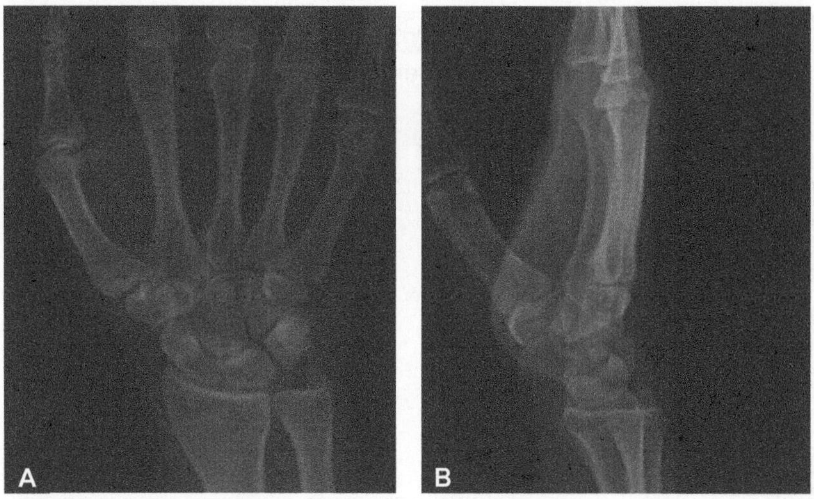

View:

Observations:

Inference:

EX. 2.18C: DETERMINATION OF AGE FROM X-RAYS

Determine the age of the male individuals from the given X-rays.

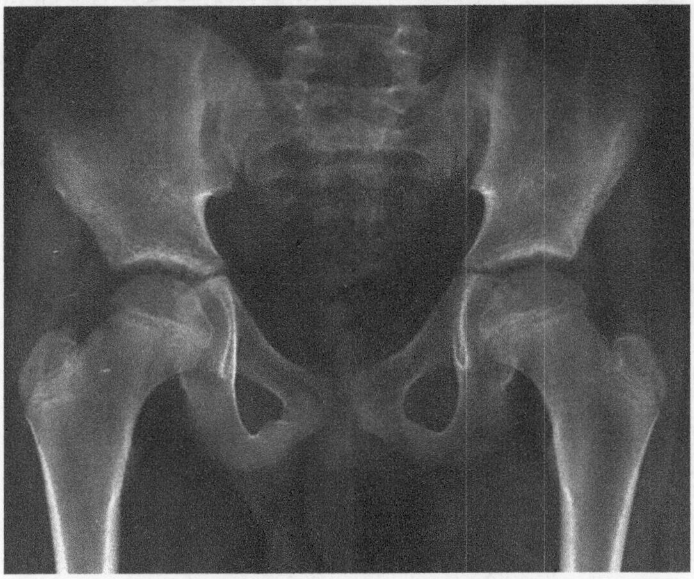

View:
Observations:
Inference:

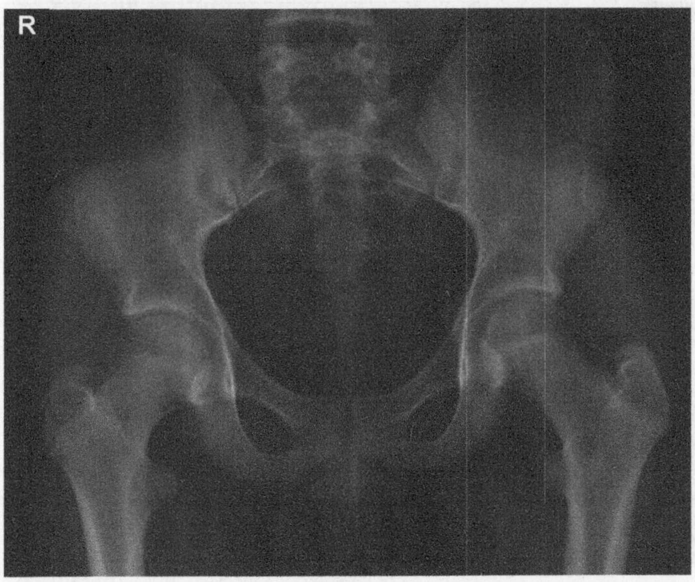

View:
Observations:
Inference:

EX. 2.18D: DETERMINATION OF AGE FROM X-RAYS

Determine the age of the male individuals from the given X-rays.

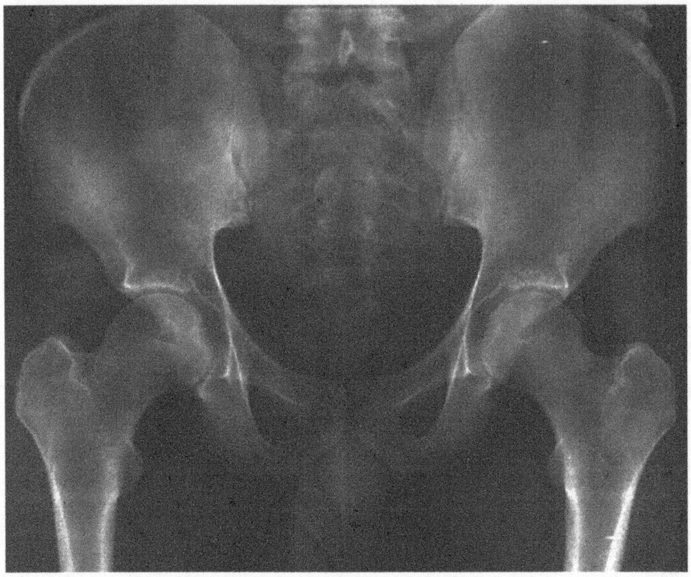

View:

Observations:

Inference:

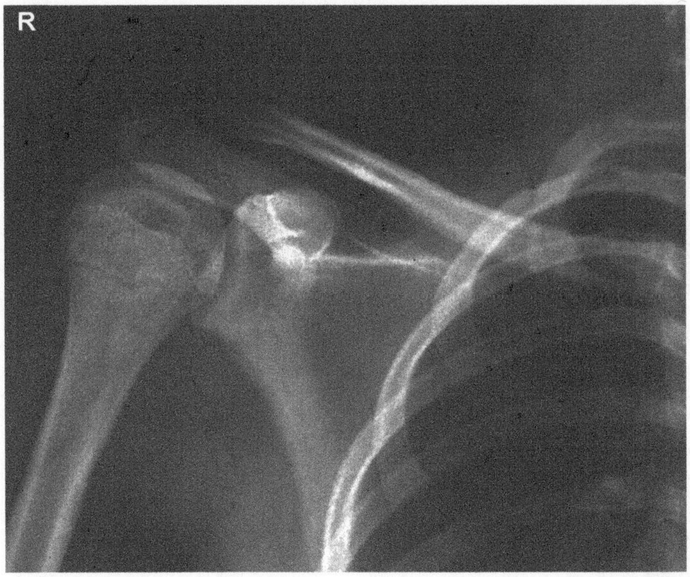

View:

Observations:

Inference:

EX. 2.19: STUDY OF FINGERPRINTS (Dactylography)

Galton System

Classification of Fingerprint Patterns

Ridge pattern (diagram)	Type	Percentage

Medicolegal Importance

Ex. 2.20: FINGERPRINT CARD

Applicant	Leave Blank	Last name NAM	First name	Middle Name	Leave Blank

Signature of person fingerprinted	ALIASES AKA	O R I	Date of birth DOB Month Day Year

Residence of person fingerprinted	Citizenship CTZ	Sex	Race	Ht.	Wt.	Eyes	Hair	Place of birth POB

Date	Signature of official Taking Fingerprints	Your No. OCA	LEAVE BLANK
Employer and address		FBI No. FBI	Class ________________
		Armed Forces No. MNU	Ref. ________________
Reason fingerprinted		Aadhar Card No. SOC	
		Miscellaneous No. MNU	

1. R. Thumb	2. R. Index	3. R. Middle	4. R. Ring	5. R. Little
6. L. Thumb	7. L. Index	8. L. Middle	9. L. Ring	10. L. Little

Left four fingers taken simultaneously	L. Thumb	R. Thumb	Right four fingers taken simultaneously

Ex. 2.21: BIOLOGICAL SPECIMEN COLLECTION FORM FOR DNA TESTING

Case Particulars

Affix a passport size signed photograph of the donor attested by medical officer in presence of I.O. or a gazetted officer.

Name ______________________

Father/ Guardian's name ______________________

Gender ____________ Age ______years ______months

Address ______________________

Medical history ______________________

____

Genetic abnormalities, if any ______________________

Blood transfusion, if any, in past three months ______________________

Organ transplantation, if any ______________________

Sample Collected for Case Examination

Case no. ____________ Date: ____________ P.S. ____________ U/S ____________

Description of sample *(Tick '✓')*

☐ Blood in EDTA ☐ Blood in FTA card

☐ Oral swab ☐ Vaginal swab ☐ ____________

Date of collection ____________ Collected by ____________

Purpose for conducting test ______________________

____

Seal impression:
(Wax covered with cellotape)

____
Signature of Medical Practioner
Name, Designation, and Seal

Declaration of the Donor/ Guardian

I, ______________________S/D/W/under guardianship of Mr/ Ms______________________ hereby declare that the biological sample (s) (______________________) thus being collected for DNA profiling is with my consent and is mine/ is of my child. I/ he/ she did not receive any blood transfusion within past three months.

Signature ____________

Name ____________

Date ____________

Left thumb impression Right thumb impression

Collection of biological sample should be preferably in presence of two witnesses.

Witness 1
Signature ____________
Name ____________
Date ____________

Witness 2
Signature ____________
Name ____________
Date ____________

EX. 2.22: EXAMINATION FOR AGE ESTIMATION IN LIVING PERSONS

A male individual Dasarath Manjhi, S/ o Jiten Manjhi was brought by the police for age estimation. He was found working in a chemical factory. He claims to be 19 years old but the police booked the owner for illegal underage employment and stated his age as 14 years. He is a resident of Madhepura, Bihar. He has no birth certificate or school leaving certificate and is illiterate. Prepare a report for the same.

Department of Forensic Medicine and Toxicology

Report No ______________________ Date and Time of Examination ______________________

Requisition from ______________________ Vide Letter No ________________ Dated ________________

Name ______________________________ S/ D/ W of ______________________________

Address ____

Gender ____________________ Occupation ____________________ Marital status ________________

Age as alleged by:

a. Individual to be examined ___________________ years

b. Police or person accompanying _______________ years

Brought by ______________________ P.C. No. ____________________ P.S. ______________________

Identification marks:

1. ____

2. ____

Informed Consent

I, ____________________________________ hereby voluntarily agree to the following: *(Tick '√' that applies)*

- ☐ Medical examination and examination of genitals and also examination of other secondary sexual characters for the purpose of age estimation.
- ☐ Radiological and dental examination for the purpose of age estimation.
- ☐ Photography for the purpose of evidence, if required.
- ☐ The report may be used for legal evidence, clinical audit, research and academic purposes.
- ☐ Inform the police and provide them the copy of this examination.*
- ☐ I have also been informed that I can refuse the whole or part of the examination and also refuse information to be given to the police. In this event, I will be responsible for any problem arising in the process of investigation and court trial.* I have been further informed that this refusal will not have any impact on the quality of treatment provided.

☐ The findings of the examination may go against me.
☐ All this has been explained to me in ______________________ language which I can understand.
* Strike out in case examination is done under the provisions of Sec. 53 CrPC

______________________ Signature/ Thumb impression ______________

______________________ Name ______________________

Signaure and name of the witness

Signature and name of the person examined or guardian (when the person is unable to give consent due to insanity or is < 12 years)

Female nurse/ attendant in presence of whom examination is conducted (if applicable)	Signature ______________________ Name ______________________

General Physical Examination

Height _________cm Weight _____________ kg Pulse ___________ / min B.P. ___________ mm Hg

Built: Poor/ Average/ Well

Secondary Sexual Characters

Male	Female
Beard/ Moustaches: Absent/ downy/ sparse/ black/ bushy	Breast development: Not developed/ developing/ well developed (Tanner stage ____________)
Pubic hair: Absent/ downy/ sparse/ black/ bushy (Tanner stage ____________)	Pubic hair: Absent/ downy/ sparse/ black/ bushy (Tanner stage ____________)
Axillary hair: Absent/ downy/ sparse/ black/ bushy	Axillary hair: Absent/ downy/ sparse/ black/ bushy
Voice: Masculine/ Feminine (Deep/ soft)	Menarche:
Adams apple: Prominent/ Not prominent	Last menstrual period:
Genitals: Scrotal/ testicular/ penile development (Tanner stage ____________)	Genitals:

Other Features

Acne ______________________ Eyes (Arcus senilis, cataract) ______________

Wrinkles on face/ skin ______________________

Other features, if any: ____

Dental Examination

Total number of teeth ____________________ Temporary ____________________ Permanent ____________________

Type of dentition: Primary/ Mixed/ Permanent

Space behind 2nd permanent molar ____________________

Dentition

	18	17	16	15	14	13	12	11	21	22	23	24	25	26	27	28	
R																	L
	48	47	46	45	44	43	42	41	31	32	33	34	35	36	37	38	

P: Permanent T: Temporary

Y: Erupted but missing X: Not erupted

Radiological examination (For appearance and fusion of centers of ossification)

Sl. No.	Part X-rayed	Observations	Inference

Orthopantomograph (OPG) findings: ____________________

____

____

OPINION

After performing general physical, dental and radiological examination, I am of the opinion that age of the subject is above ______________ years and below ______________ years of age.

(____________________)

Place ______________

Date ______________

Signature of Medical Officer

Name, Designation and Seal

Received Report No. ____________________

Name ____________________ P.C. No ______________ P.S. ______________

Signature and date

Requisition for Radiological Examination for Estimation of Age

Department of Forensic Medicine and Toxicology

Ref. No ____________ Date ____________

To

The Professor/ Medical Officer I/ C

Department of Radiology

____

Subject: Estimation of age of ________________________________

Dear Sir/ Madam,

Ref. Requisition from ________________________ dated ____________

I request that radiographs of the subject may be taken as indicated below.

Sl. No.	Region	View

The subject bears the following identification marks:

1. ________________________________
2. ________________________________

I request you that the X-ray plates may be sent to me at the earliest.

Yours faithfully

____

Signature of Medical Officer

Place ____________

Date ____________

Name, Designation and Seal

Ex. 2.23: EXAMINATION OF SKELETAL REMAINS

A primary school student while playing in the mountains discovered a skeletonized femur, and reported this to his mother. During a search of the vicinity, the right femur, right tibia, pelvis and skull (depressed fracture present in right parietal area) along with mandible (2 mandibular and 7 maxillary teeth were present, rest missing) were discovered. The police sent it to you to determine whether they belong to the same person (since the sites of discovery differed) and whether identity and cause of death could be established. Draft a report for the same.

Department of Forensic Medicine and Toxicology

____

Report No. ______________ Date ______________

Requisition from ______________________________ Dated ______________

Brought by ______________________ P.C. No. ______________ P.S. ________

Examination Findings

A. Description [List of bone(s) received]

☐ Complete skeleton ☐ Partial skeleton ☐ Fragmentary remains ☐ Only skull

B. Condition of skeleton

☐ Cracking ☐ Brittle ☐ Breaks ☐ Cut marks ☐ Gnaw marks

☐ Exfoliation ☐ Warping ☐ Insect damage ☐ Soil adhering ☐ Staining

C. Origin of the bone (whether the bones are human or not?)

a. Anatomical characteristics
b. Microscopic examination
c. Analysis of bone ash
d. Precipitin test

D. Whether they belong to one or more individuals?

a. Number, side and size of the bones
b. Age and sex
c. Morphological similarities
d. Use of short wave UV light
e. X-ray comparison of trabecular pattern
f. Neutron activation analysis

E. The stature of the individual to whom the bones belonged.
Multiplication factor or regression analysis

F. The race of the individual to whom the bones belonged.
Indices and racial peculiarities

G. The sex of the individual to whom the bones belonged.
  a. General characteristics
  b. Specific changes in the individual bone
  c. Examination of the soft parts, if available

H. The age of the individual to whom the bones belonged.
  a. Dental status, if skull or mandible is available
  b. Ossification data
  c. Secondary changes in the bones like closure of skull sutures, bony joint surfaces, etc.

I. Whether the bones have been cut, sawn, gnawed by animals or burnt?

J. Any other feature(s) that may help in identification of the individual.
  a. Congenital abnormalities or deformities
  b. Acquired peculiarities – injuries, fractures, etc.
  c. Determination of the blood group from the marrow/ tooth pulp
  d. Radiological examination.

Opinion

i. From the above findings, I am opinion that the bone(s) belong to ______________________ origin

of ______________________ sex and aged about ______________________ .

ii. Cause of death
  a. Any injuries/ fracture
  b. Foreign body (bullet, pellets or any piece of weapon)
  c Chemical analysis for poisoning
  d. Neutron activation analysis

iii. Time since death
  a. State of soft tissue, if available
  b. Changes due to putrefaction
  c. Stages of healing in case of fracture

____

Signature of Medical Officer
Name, Designation and Seal

Received Report No. ______________________, bundle of bones, packed and sealed along with the sample seal.

Name ______________________ P.C. No ______________________ P.S. ______________________

Signature and date

Ex. 2.23A: EXAMINATION OF SKELETAL REMAINS (Details)

Adult Skeletal Inventory

Report No. _______________

Codes
P = Present (Complete)
A = Absent
F = Fragment

Cranial

Bone		Bone	
Parietal		Frontal	
Temporal		Occipital	
Maxilla		Sphenoid	
Nasal		Vomer	
Zygomatic		Ethmoid	
Lacrimal		Hyoid	
Palatine		Cricoid	
Mandible		Thyroid	
Orbit			

Right ribs [ ]

Left ribs [ ]

Axial

C1		T6	
C2		T7	
C3		T8	
C4		T9	
C5		T10	
C6		T11	
C7		T12	
T1		L1	
T2		L2	
T3		L3	
T4		L4	
T5		L5	

Right Appendicular

Bone	
Humerus	
Radius	
Ulna	
Femur	
Tibia	
Fibula	

Left Appendicular

Bone	
Humerus	
Radius	
Ulna	
Femur	
Tibia	
Fibula	

Right Appendicular

Bone	
Ilium	
Ischium	
Pubis	
Scapula	
Clavicle	
Patella	

Left Appendicular

Bone	
Ilium	
Ischium	
Pubis	
Scapula	
Clavicle	
Patella	

Bone	
Sternum	
Coccyx	
Sacrum	

Teeth	
Incisors	
Canines	
Premolars	
Molars	

Extremities

Right	1	2	3	4	5
Metacarpals					
Metatarsals					

Left	1	2	3	4	5
Metacarpals					
Metatarsals					

	Scaphoid	Lunate	Triquetral	Pisiform	Trapezium	Trapezoid	Capitate	Hamate	Sesmoid
Right									
Left									
	Talus	Calcaneus	1st Cun	2nd Cun	3rd Cun	Navicular	Cuboid		Sesmoid
Right									
Left									

Hand Proximal phalanges ☐ Middle phalanges ☐ Distal phalanges ☐

Foot Proximal phalanges ☐ Middle phalanges ☐ Distal phalanges ☐

EX. 2.23B: EXAMINATION OF SKELETAL REMAINS (Details)

Report No. ____________

Fill in skeletal elements present and record notes along side.

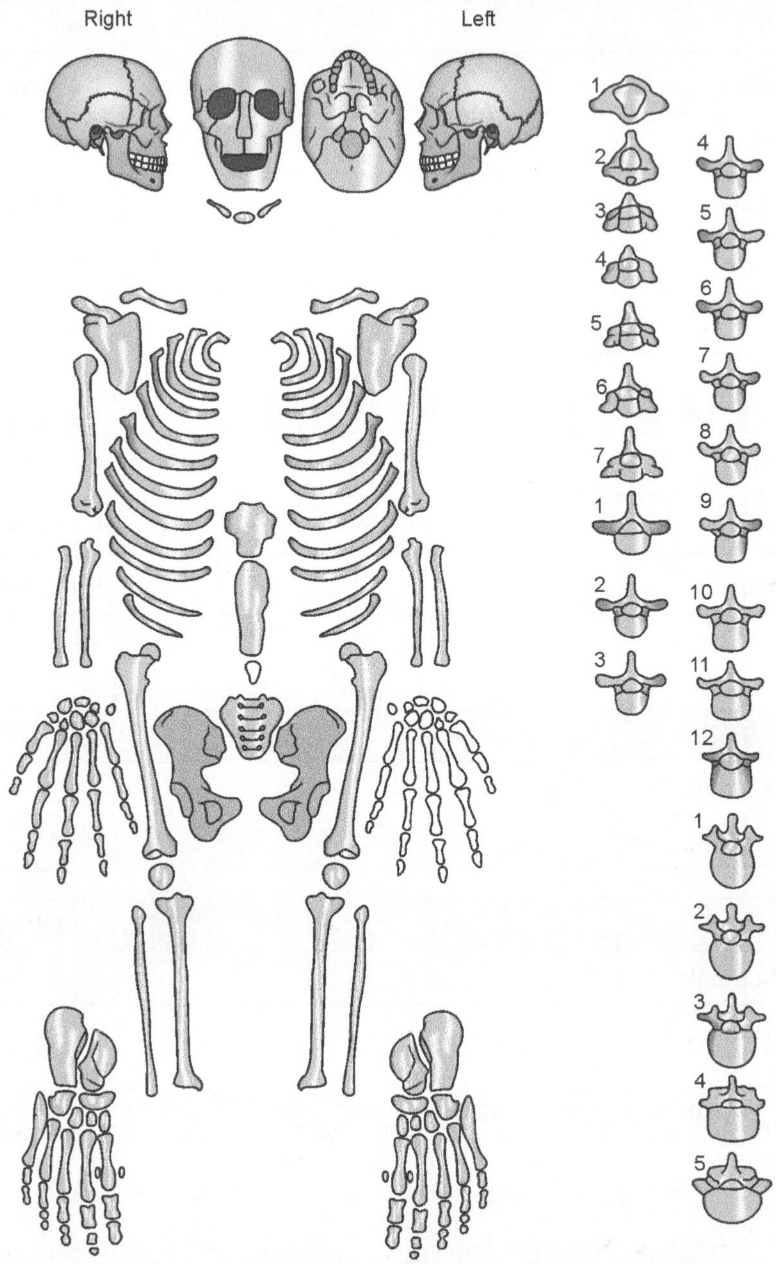

Additional observations:

Ex. 2.23C: EXAMINATION OF SKELETAL REMAINS (Details)

Age and Sex Assessment (Adult)

Report No.________
Age:________
Sex:________

AGE

PELVIC	Left	Right
Pubic Symphysis		
Todd (1–10)	____	____
Suchey-Brooks (1–6)	____	____
Auricular Surface		
Lovejoy et al (1–8)	____	____

POSTCRANIAL: Epiphyseal Union*

Clavicle	Sternal	epiphysis	____
Vertebral	Cervical	superior	____
Annular	Thoracic	inferior	____
		superior	____
	Lumbar	inferior	____
Sacrum	S1/ S2 fusion		____
Innominate	Iliac crest		____

Estimated Age:	Subadult (12–20 years)	____
	Young Adult (20–35 years)	____
	Middle Adult (35–50 years)	____
	Old Adult (50+ years)	____

CRANIAL		Suture Closure*	
External	1.	Midlambdoid	____
Cranial	2.	Lambda	____
Vault	3.	Obelion	____
	4.	Anterior Sagittal	____
	5.	Bregma	____
	6.	Midcoronal	____
	7.	Pterion	____
	8.	Sphenofrontal	____
	9.	Inf. Sphenotemporal	____
	10.	Sup. Sphenotemporal	____
Palatine	11.	Incisive Suture	____
	12.	Anterior Median	____
	13.	Posterior Median	____
	14.	Transverse Palatine	____
Internal	15.	Sagittal	____
Cranial	16.	Left Lambdoid	____
Vault	17.	Left Coronal	____

**Suture and Epiphysis Codes*
0 = Open
1 = Minimal
2 = Significant
3 = Complete

Observations:

SEX

PELVIC	Left	Right
Ventral Arc (1–3)	____	____
Subpubic Concavity (1–3)	____	____
Ischiopubic Ramus Ridge (1–3)	____	____
Greater Sciatic Notch (1–5)	____	____
Preauricular Sulcus (0–4)	____	____
Estimated Sex, Pelvis (1–5):	____ =	____

CRANIAL	
Nuchal Crest (1–5)	____
Mastoid Process (1–5)	____
Supraorbital Margin (1–5)	____
Glabella (1–5)	____
Mental Eminence (–-5)	____
Estimated Sex, Skull (1–5):	____ = ____

Observations:

Ex. 2.23D: EXAMINATION OF SKELETAL REMAINS (Details)

Age Assessment (Juvenile)

Report No. ____________

Stage of Union
0 = Open
1 = Minimal
2 = Complete

Epiphyseal Union

Element	Epiphysis	Stage of union left	Stage of union right
Scapula	Coracoid	______	______
	Acromium	______	______
Clavicle	Sternal	______	______
Humerus	Head	______	______
	Distal	______	______
	Med. epicondyle	______	______
Radius	Proximal	______	______
	Distal	______	______
Ulna	Proximal	______	______
	Distal	______	______
Pelvis	Iliac crest	______	______
	Ischial tuberosity	______	______
Femur	Head	______	______
	Greater trochanter	______	______
	Lesser trochanter	______	______
	Distal	______	______
Tibia	Proximal	______	______
	Distal	______	______
Fibula	Proximal	______	______
	Distal	______	______
Metacarpals	Proximal (1st)	______	
	Distal (2–5)	______	
Metatarsals	Proximal (1st)	______	
	Distal (2–5)	______	
C. Phalanges	Proximal	______	
T. Phalanges	Proximal	______	

Primary Ossification Centers

Element	Area of union	Stage of union
Innominate	Ilium-pubis	______
	Ischium-pubis	______
	Ischium-ilium	______
Sacrum	1–2	______
	2–3	______
	3–4	______
	4–5	______
Cervical vertebrae		
	Neural arches to each other	______
	Neural arches to centrum	______
Thoracic vertebrae		
	Neural arches to each other	______
	Neural arches to centrum	______
Lumbar vertebrae		
	Neural arches to each other	______
	Neural arches to centrum	______
Cranium		
	Basilar suture	______
Occipital		
	Lateral–squama	______
	Basilar-lateral	______
Mandibular Symphysis		______
Metopic Suture		______

Age Assessment

	Age class	Age range in months or years	
Fetus	________	lunar months	________
Infant (birth –1 year)	________	months/ years	________
Child (1–12 years)	________	years	________
Subadult (12–20 years)	________	years	________

Comments (criteria used for age assessment):

Ex. 2.23E: EXAMINATION OF SKELETAL REMAINS (Details)

Dental Examination of Human Remains

Site of discovery: ______	Report No.: ______
Condition of remains: ______	Body No. : ______
Cause of death: ______	Sex: ______

11			21
12			22
13			23
14			24
15			25
16			26
17			27
18			28

18 17 16 15 14 13 12 11 21 22 23 24 25 26 27 28

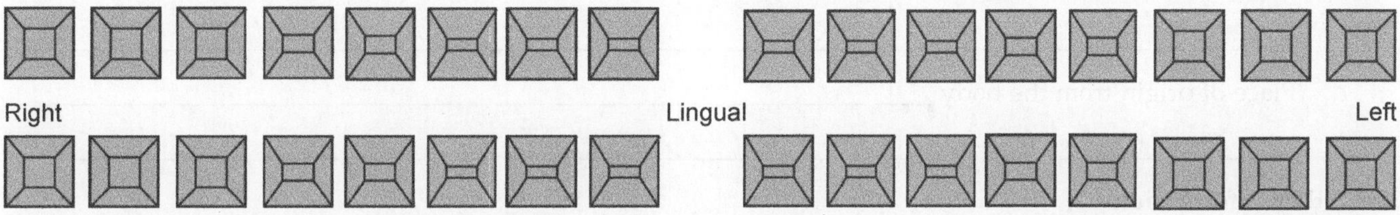

Right Lingual Left

48 47 46 45 44 43 42 41 31 32 33 34 35 36 37 38

48			38
47			37
46			36
45			35
44			34
43			33
42			34
41			31

Occlusion:		Crowns:		Bridges:		Smoker:
Dentures:	P/ U F/ U P/ L F/ L	Material: Marks:		Teeth:	Type: Mould: Shade:	
Maxillofacial Prosthesis: Implants:				Clasps:	Type:	
Radiographs: Photographs	Bw. Clinical	Pa:	Occ.	Lat. Portrait	AP	OPC
Special Treatments		Endo	Perio	Ortho	Oral Surgery	C and B

Ex. 2.24: EXAMINATION OF HAIR

A. Structure of Hair ____________________

____

Hair or fiber ____________________

____

B. Source of Hair

a. Human or Animal Hair ____________________

Medullary Index ____________________

b. Racial differences ____________________

____

c. Male or Female Hair ____________________

____

d. Place of origin from the body ____________________

____

C. Other Information

a. Age of the person ____________________

____

b. Any alteration/ disease ____________________

____

c. Naturally removed or traumatic ____________________

____

d. Toxicological information ____________________

____

D. Medicolegal Importance

____

____

____

____

____

Difference between Hair and Fiber

Feature	Hair	Fiber

Difference between Human Hair and Animal Hair

Feature	Hair	Fiber

EX. 2.25: EXAMINATION OF SEMINAL STAINS

A. **Purpose of Examination** ____________________

____

____

B. **Methods of Examination**

i. Physical Examination: (quality, viscosity, odor, solubility, appearance) ____________________

____

____

ii. Examination under U-V light ____________________

____

iii. **CHEMICAL EXAMINATION**

a. **Florence Test**

Procedure ____________________

____

____

Observations ____________________

____

b. **Barberio's Test**

Procedure ____________________

____

____

Observations ____________________

____

c. **Acid Phosphatase Test (Brentamine Fast Blue Test)**

Procedure ____________________

____

____

Observations ____________________

____

iv. **Microscopic Examination**

Procedure ______________________________

Observations ______________________________

v. **Other Staining Methods and Noncellular Semen Markers**

a. Christmas tree stain ______________________________

b. Acid phosphatase test (quantitative) ______________________________

c. Prostate specific antigen (p30) ______________________________

d. Semenogelin ______________________________

vi. **Species origin** ______________________________

vii. **Individualization of Seminal stains**

a. Blood group --*Secretors/ Nonsecretors* ______________________________

b. Enzyme typing ______________________________

c. DNA profiling ______________________________

C. **Medicolegal Issues**

____

EX. 2.26: EXAMINATION OF BLOODSTAINS

A. **Purpose of Examination** ________________________________

B. **Methods of Examination**

a. Physical Examination ________________________________

b. Chemical Examination **(Phenolphthalein Test or Kastle-Meyer Test)**

Procedure ________________________________

Observations ________________________________

c. Microscopic or Microchemical Examination

i. **Hemochromogen Crystal Test (Takayama Test)**

Procedure ________________________________

Observations ________________________________

ii. **Hemin Crystal Test (Teichmann's Test)**

Procedure ________________________________

Observations ________________________________

d. **Microscopic Examination** (Human or Animal Blood)

e. **Spectroscopic Examination**

f. **Biological/ Serological Examination**

i. *Precipitin Test*

ii. *Blood Grouping*

C. Medicolegal Issues

EX. 2.27: FETAL EXAMINATION FOR INTRAUTERINE AGE

Age (in months)	Features/ Findings

Rule of Hasse ____________________

____

____

NOTES

NOTES

NOTES

UNIT III

Study of Museum Specimens and Slides

EX. 3.1: STUDY OF WEAPONS OF OFFENCE (BLUNT)

Name, describe and make a labeled diagram of the weapon and mention the injuries possible with it.

Labeled diagram	Description and injuries possible

EX. 3.2: STUDY OF WEAPONS OF OFFENCE (Sharp Cutting)

Name, describe and make a labeled diagram of the weapon and mention the injuries possible with it.

Labeled diagram	Description and injuries possible

EX. 3.3: STUDY OF WEAPONS OF OFFENCE (Sharp Heavy Cutting)

Name, describe and make a labeled diagram of the weapon and mention the injuries possible with it.

Labeled diagram	Description and injuries possible

EX. 3.4: STUDY OF WEAPONS OF OFFENCE (Pointed)

Name, describe and make a labeled diagram of the weapon and mention the injuries possible with it.

Labeled diagram	Description and injuries possible

EX. 3.5: STUDY OF WEAPONS OF OFFENCE (Firearms)

Name, describe and make a labeled diagram of the weapon and mention the injuries possible with it.

Labeled diagram	Description and injuries possible

EX. 3.6: STUDY OF WEAPONS OF OFFENCE (Others/Mixed)

Name, describe and make a labeled diagram of the weapon and mention the injuries possible with it.

Labeled diagram	Description and injuries possible

EX. 3.7A: STUDY OF MUSEUM SPECIMENS (Wet)

Specimen 1

Identification:

Observation:

Opinion:

Medicolegal significance:

Specimen 2

Identification:

Observation:

Opinion:

Medicolegal significance:

Specimen 3

Identification:

Observation:

Opinion:

Medicolegal significance:

Specimen 4

Identification:

Observation:

Opinion:

Medicolegal significance:

EX. 3.7B: STUDY OF MUSEUM SPECIMENS (Wet)

Specimen 5
Identification: Observation: Opinion: Medicolegal significance:
Specimen 6
Identification: Observation: Opinion: Medicolegal significance:
Specimen 7
Identification: Observation: Opinion: Medicolegal significance:
Specimen 8
Identification: Observation: Opinion: Medicolegal significance:

EX. 3.7C: STUDY OF MUSEUM SPECIMENS (Wet)

Specimen 9
Identification:
Observation:
Opinion:
Medicolegal significance:
Specimen 10
Identification:
Observation:
Opinion:
Medicolegal significance:
Specimen 11
Identification:
Observation:
Opinion:
Medicolegal significance:
Specimen 12
Identification:
Observation:
Opinion:
Medicolegal significance:

Ex. 3.7D: STUDY OF MUSEUM SPECIMENS (Wet)

Specimen 13
Identification: Observation: Opinion: Medicolegal significance:

Specimen 14
Identification: Observation: Opinion: Medicolegal significance:

Specimen 15
Identification: Observation: Opinion: Medicolegal significance:

Specimen 16
Identification: Observation: Opinion: Medicolegal significance:

EX. 3.8A: STUDY OF MODELS

Model 1
Identification:
Observation:
Opinion:
Medicolegal significance:
Model 2
Identification:
Observation:
Opinion:
Medicolegal significance:
Model 3
Identification:
Observation:
Opinion:
Medicolegal significance:
Model 4
Identification:
Observation:
Opinion:
Medicolegal significance:

EX. 3.8B: STUDY OF MODELS

Model 5
Identification: Observation: Opinion: Medicolegal significance:
Model 6
Identification: Observation: Opinion: Medicolegal significance:
Model 7
Identification: Observation: Opinion: Medicolegal significance:
Model 8
Identification: Observation: Opinion: Medicolegal significance:

EX. 3.9A: STUDY OF PHOTOGRAPHS

Photograph 1
Identification: Observation: Opinion: Medicolegal significance:

Photograph 2
Identification: Observation: Opinion: Medicolegal significance:

Photograph 3
Identification: Observation: Opinion: Medicolegal significance:

Photograph 4
Identification: Observation: Opinion: Medicolegal significance:

EX.3.9B: STUDY OF PHOTOGRAPHS

Photograph 5
Identification: Observation: Opinion: Medicolegal significance:
Photograph 6
Identification: Observation: Opinion: Medicolegal significance:
Photograph 7
Identification: Observation: Opinion: Medicolegal significance:
Photograph 8
Identification: Observation: Opinion: Medicolegal significance:

EX. 3.9C: STUDY OF PHOTOGRAPHS

Photograph 9
Identification: Observation: Opinion: Medicolegal significance:
Photograph 10
Identification: Observation: Opinion: Medicolegal significance:
Photograph 11
Identification: Observation: Opinion: Medicolegal significance:
Photograph 12
Identification: Observation: Opinion: Medicolegal significance:

EX. 3.10A: STUDY OF MICROSCOPIC SLIDES

Slide 1

Identification:

Observation:

Opinion:

Medicolegal significance:

Slide 2

Identification:

Observation:

Opinion:

Medicolegal significance:

Slide 3

Identification:

Observation:

Opinion:

Medicolegal significance:

Slide 4

Identification:

Observation:

Opinion:

Medicolegal significance:

EX. 3.10B: STUDY OF MICROSCOPIC SLIDES

Slide 5

Identification:

Observation:

Opinion:

Medicolegal significance:

Slide 6

Identification:

Observation:

Opinion:

Medicolegal significance:

Slide 7

Identification:

Observation:

Opinion:

Medicolegal significance:

Slide 8

Identification:

Observation:

Opinion:

Medicolegal significance:

EX. 3.11: STUDY OF TOXICOLOGICAL

Sl. No.	Name of Poison	Physical Characteristics and Salient Clinical Features

SPECIMENS (Corrosives)

Fatal Dose	Fatal Period	Management	Postmortem Findings	Medicolegal Significance

EX. 3.12: STUDY OF TOXICOLOGICAL

Metallic and

Sl. No.	Name of Poison	Physical Characteristics and Salient Clinical Features

SPECIMENS (Irritant Inorganic Poisons)

Non-metallic Poisons

Fatal Dose	Fatal Period	Management	Postmortem Findings	Medicolegal Significance

EX. 3.13: STUDY OF TOXICOLOGICAL

Plant

Sl. No.	Name of Poison	Physical Characteristics and Salient Clinical Features	Active Principles

SPECIMENS (Irritant Organic Poisons)

Poisons

Fatal Dose	Fatal Period	Management	Postmortem Findings	Medicolegal Significance

Ex. 3.14 STUDY OF TOXICOLOGICAL

Animal

Sl. No.	Name of Poison	Physical Characteristics and Salient Clinical Features	Toxic/Active Principles

SPECIMENS (Irritant Organic Poisons)

Poisons

Fatal Dose	Fatal Period	Management	Postmortem Findings	Medicolegal Significance

EX. 3.15 STUDY OF TOXICOLOGICAL

Somniferous

Sl. No.	Name of Poison	Physical Characteristics and Salient Clinical Features	Active Principles

SPECIMENS (Neurotic Cerebral Poisons)

Poisons

Fatal Dose	Fatal Period	Management	Postmortem Findings	Medicolegal Significance

EX. 3.16: STUDY OF TOXICOLOGICAL

Inebriant

Sl. No.	Name of Poison	Physical Characteristics and Salient Clinical Features

SPECIMENS (Neurotic Cerebral Poisons)

Poisons

Fatal Dose	Fatal Period	Management	Postmortem Findings	Medicolegal Significance

EX. 3.17: STUDY OF TOXICOLOGICAL

Deliriant

Sl. No.	Name of Poison	Physical Characteristics and Salient Clinical Features	Active Principles

SPECIMENS (Neurotic Cerebral Poisons)

Poisons

Fatal Dose	Fatal Period	Management	Postmortem Findings	Medicolegal Significance

EX. 3.18: STUDY OF TOXICOLOGICAL

Sl. No.	Name of Poison	Physical Characteristics and Salient Clinical Features	Active Principles

SPECIMENS (Spinal and Peripheral Poisons)

Fatal Dose	Fatal Period	Management	Postmortem Findings	Medicolegal Significance

EX. 3.19: STUDY OF TOXICOLOGICAL

Sl. No.	Name of Poison	Physical Characteristics and Salient Clinical Features	Active Principles

SPECIMENS (Cardiac and Asphyxiant Poisons)

Fatal Dose	Fatal Period	Management	Postmortem Findings	Medicolegal Significance

EX. 3.20: STUDY OF TOXICOLOGICAL

Agrochemical

Sl. No.	Name of Poison	Physical Characteristics and Salient Clinical Features

SPECIMENS (Miscellaneous Poisons)

Poisons

Fatal Dose	Fatal Period	Management	Postmortem Findings	Medicolegal Significance

EX. 3.21: STUDY OF TOXICOLOGICAL

Drugs of Dependence, Street/ Designer Drugs

Sl. No.	Name of Poison	Physical Characteristics and Salient Clinical Features

SPECIMENS (Miscellaneous Poisons)

Hydrocarbons, Poisonous Foods

Fatal Dose	Fatal Period	Management	Postmortem Findings	Medicolegal Significance

NOTES

NOTES

NOTES

Medicolegal Report/ Injury Report

Medicolegal case: A case of injury or ailment where the medical practitioner after history taking and clinical examination considers that investigations by law enforcement agencies are necessary to ascertain circumstances of the causation of the said injury or ailment.

Medicolegal Report

A medicolegal report (MLR) is a report on the condition of a patient, solicited for legal purposes which gives the medical expert's findings, diagnosis, prognosis and opinion. It is a structured and formal mode of communication between the doctor and the legal system.

The format should help the medical officer to give a comprehensive report that clearly separates the facts from the opinions, and provides a basis for the opinion stated.

Guidelines for Writing a MLR

- Medicolegal injury cases should be examined without delay at anytime of the day or night.
- All details of examination of the injured person, whether admitted into hospital or treated in OPD have to be entered in a Medicolegal Register.
- This register is a confidential record and should be in safe custody of the medical officer. It has to be produced in the court of law, if asked for.
- The particulars are entered in the injury report by the medical practitioner in his/ her own handwriting (at some places computerized reports are being issued).
- Cutting/ overwriting should be avoided as much as possible and all corrections should be properly initialed. It should be corrected legibly by lining out with a single line, initializing with date.
- The report should be comprehensive without being unnecessarily wordy and over-inclusive.
- The report is usually addressed to the police and the lawyers who are not themselves experts in medical field. Hence, the report should be written in clear and understandable English, with as little use of technical terms and professional jargon as possible.
- Abbreviations should be avoided—write all the entries including the medical terms in a full form. Symbol '#' used to denote a fracture in medical notes should not be used in MLRs. 'Contused lacerated wound' instead of 'c.l.w' is to be written.
- During examination of a female subject by a male doctor, a nurse/ female attendant MUST BE PRESENT.
- The report should always be signed by the medical practitioner to authenticate it along with date, his/ her full name, designation, registration number, current employment and qualifications at appropriate place.

Date and time of examination

- Every medicolegal report must include the date and time of examination.
- It is important to include the time when the examination began and ended, as this may support the contention that the examination was a complete and thorough one.

Consent

Before starting of examination, informed written consent from the patient or the legal guardian is to be taken in writing (preferably in presence of disinterested witness).

Identification marks

- It is better to note down at least 2 identification marks.
- If only one identification mark is recorded, there may be a chance of loss of one mark due to any reason—scarification or amputation of that part; and during subsequent examination it may cause difficulty in identification.

The marks used for identification:

- Congenital marks—birth marks, moles, nevus, supernumerary teeth/ fingers, cleft palate, etc.
- Acquired marks—scar, tattoo, deformities, malunited fractures, etc.

History

'Alleged' short history of the case is noted as stated by the patient/ persons accompanying the patient. If the patient is conscious and able to speak, history of the incidence is recorded from the patient. If the patient is unconscious, history of the incidence is then taken from the persons accompanying the patient. Questions should include:

a. Date and time of infliction of injury.
b. How the injury was sustained, if assaulted, number of persons involved.
c. Whether any weapon was used, if so what type of weapon; if it was hard, blunt or sharp cutting or pointed, etc.
d. Whether any first aid/ treatment was given at any place?

If serious, dying declaration is recorded as required.

General physical examination

- Consciousness, orientation, pulse, temperature, blood pressure, reaction of pupils to light.
- Size of the victim, i.e. stature, weight and development (in case of children/ adolescents).

Examination of injuries

A few basic items are also essential prior to examination: a hand lens, measuring scale and a torch, and the injuries are described as given in Table 4.1. The injuries should be highlighted in a separate body diagram too.

Table 4.1: Describing features of physical injuries

Feature	Notes
Type	All injuries, i.e. abrasion, contusion, laceration, incised wound, etc. observed, even insignificant, should be noted. A lens should be used to get an accurate idea of the nature of edges, ends and floor of the wound.
Site	Record the anatomical position of the wound(s) with reference to some landmark, e.g. midline, bony structure, umbilicus.
Size	The dimensions of the wound(s) should be measured and never guessed, and amount of blood extravasated should be measured.
Shape	Describe the shape of the wound(s) (e.g. linear, curved, irregular, circular, oval or triangular) and also the beveling of the edges.
Surrounds	Note the condition of the surrounding or the nearby tissues (e.g. bruised, swollen).

Contd...

Contd...

Color	Observation of color is particularly relevant when describing bruises and abrasions.
Course	Comment on the apparent direction of the force applied (e.g. in abrasions and incised wounds) viz. horizontal, vertical or oblique with regard to anatomical position of the body.
Contents	Note the presence of any foreign material in the wound(s) (e.g. dirt, glass).
Age	Comment on any evidence of healing. Note that accurate ageing is impossible and great caution is required when commenting on this aspect.
Borders	The characteristics of the edges of the wound(s) may provide a clue as to the weapon used.
Depth	Give an indication of the depth of the wound(s); this may have to be an estimate.

Advice

- It is appropriate to mention the investigations, procedures and management of the patient.
- In all injuries, when fracture of a bone is suspected, an X-ray should be done for confirmation.

Samples and Specimens

- Samples and specimens collected should be properly identified, sealed and labeled.
- They should be kept in safe custody and handed over to the I.O. of the case.
- Specimens once collected, loss/ destruction of evidence is a punishable offence.
- All evidence collected should be mentioned in MLR to establish the chain of custody in a court of law subsequently.

Opinion

What was the type of weapon used?

- In many cases, examination of the wound and clothing give fairly definite information about the kind of weapon (hard blunt object/ impact or sharp/ blunt edged/ pointed instrument or object).
- With stabs and incised wound, there is not much difficulty.

What was the nature of the injury?

- Opinion is given as to whether the injuries were simple or grievous in nature.
- Against each injury, it should be noted whether it is simple or grievous.
- Injured person must be kept under observation, if nature of particular injury cannot be made out at the time of examination, e.g. head injury or abdominal injury.
- The initial or provisional report should be made available immediately.
- A subsequent report (supplementary report) should be given, once the investigation results become available—reflects the final conclusions drawn from the examination findings.
- Whether an injury is simple or grievous is decided on the basis of *status of injury at the time of infliction* and not after medical/ surgical intervention.

What is the time passed since infliction of the injury?

Opinion is based on the state of healing of the injuries as was recorded in the column of examination of the injuries.

What was the manner of infliction of injury?

The history, clinical examination and findings on investigations and examination, all are considered together to opine whether the injuries sustained are consistent with alleged history [fall or road traffic accident (or any other accident) or assault].

EX. 4.1: BASIC DEFINITIONS

A. Injury (as per Sec. ______________ IPC) ______________________________

____

B. Hurt (as per Sec. ___________ IPC) ______________________________

____

C. Simple injury ____

____

D. Grievous hurt (as per Sec. ____________ IPC)

Clauses	Description

E. Dangerous injuries ____

____

____

F. Dangerous weapons or means (as per Sec. _____________ and Sec. ________________ IPC) _____________

____

____

____

EX. 4.2: MEDICOLEGAL CASE INFORMATION

Department of Emergency Medicine

____

Time______________ AM/ PM Date________________

To

The Officer Incharge

______________Police Station,

___________ City/ District

Subject: Police information regarding a Medicolegal Case reporting to the Emergency Department

Sir,

This is to inform you that patient Mr/ Ms ________________________________

S/ D/ W of ________________________ aged about __________ years and resident of

____(complete address)

has been brought to the emergency with alleged history of________________________,

brought by ____________________ and alleged to have occurred at ______________

________________________________ Police Station ______________.

He/ she is being treated/ discharged/ left against medical advice/ expired in the emergency/ OPD/ __________

ward of ________________ Hospital (Central Registration No. __________________).

Date and time of admission ____________________ Diagnosis ____________________

This information is being sent through ________________ Designation ________________.

This information is for further necessary action please.

Thanking you.

Signature of the Medical Officer
Name, Designation and Seal

Time and date of receiving the information at the police post ______________

Signature of the Police Officer______________

Name (in capital letters) ______________

Seal of the Police Post

EX. 4.3: BROUGHT DEAD CASE INFORMATION

Department of Emergency Medicine

Time_____________ AM/ PM   Date______________

To

The Officer Incharge

______________Police Station,

___________ City/ District

Subject: Police information regarding a Brought Dead Case reporting to the Emergency Department

Sir,

This is to inform you that patient Mr/ Ms ____

S/ D/ W of ___________________________ aged about ______________ years and resident of

____(complete address)

has been brought dead to the emergency with alleged history of_____________________________,

brought by _______________________ and alleged to have occurred at ____________________

____________________________________ Police Station ______________________.

This information is being sent through __________________ Designation __________________.

This information is for further necessary action please.

Thanking you.

Signature of the Medical Officer
Name, Designation and Seal

Time and date of receiving the information at the police post ________________

Signature of the Police Officer________________

Name (in capital letters) ________________

Seal of the Police Post

EX. 4.4: MEDICOLEGAL REPORT I

Ankur Ranawat, a 38-year-old male while going to office on his motorcycle was hit by a car coming from opposite side at 10.00 AM. He was rushed to the emergency department of your hospital in unconscious state. Prepare a medicolegal report showing one simple and two grievous injuries on his person.

CR. No. ________________ MLR No. ________________

Name ______________________ S/ D/ W of ______________________ Age ______ Gender ______

Residence ______________________ Occupation ____________ Police Station ____________

Brought by ______________________ Date and Time of Examination ________________

(If relative/ friend — Name, address and signature)

Date and time of admission ________________

No. and date of police docket ________________

No. and name of constable ________________

Articles handed over to the police

CONSENT

I am willing for my medicolegal examination.
I have not been examined earlier.
I will show all my injuries on my person.
I have been explained that the result of the examination may go in my favor or against me.

Signature/ Thumb Impression of patient/ guardian

History

General Condition (Vitals)

Particulars of Injuries

Identification Marks

1. ______________________
2. ______________________

1. Nature of Injuries ________________
   (Simple/ grievous)
   ____
2. Probable duration of injuries ________________
   ____

Kind of weapon used

____

Signature of the Doctor
Name, Designation and Seal

Date __________ MLR No. __________ CR No. __________

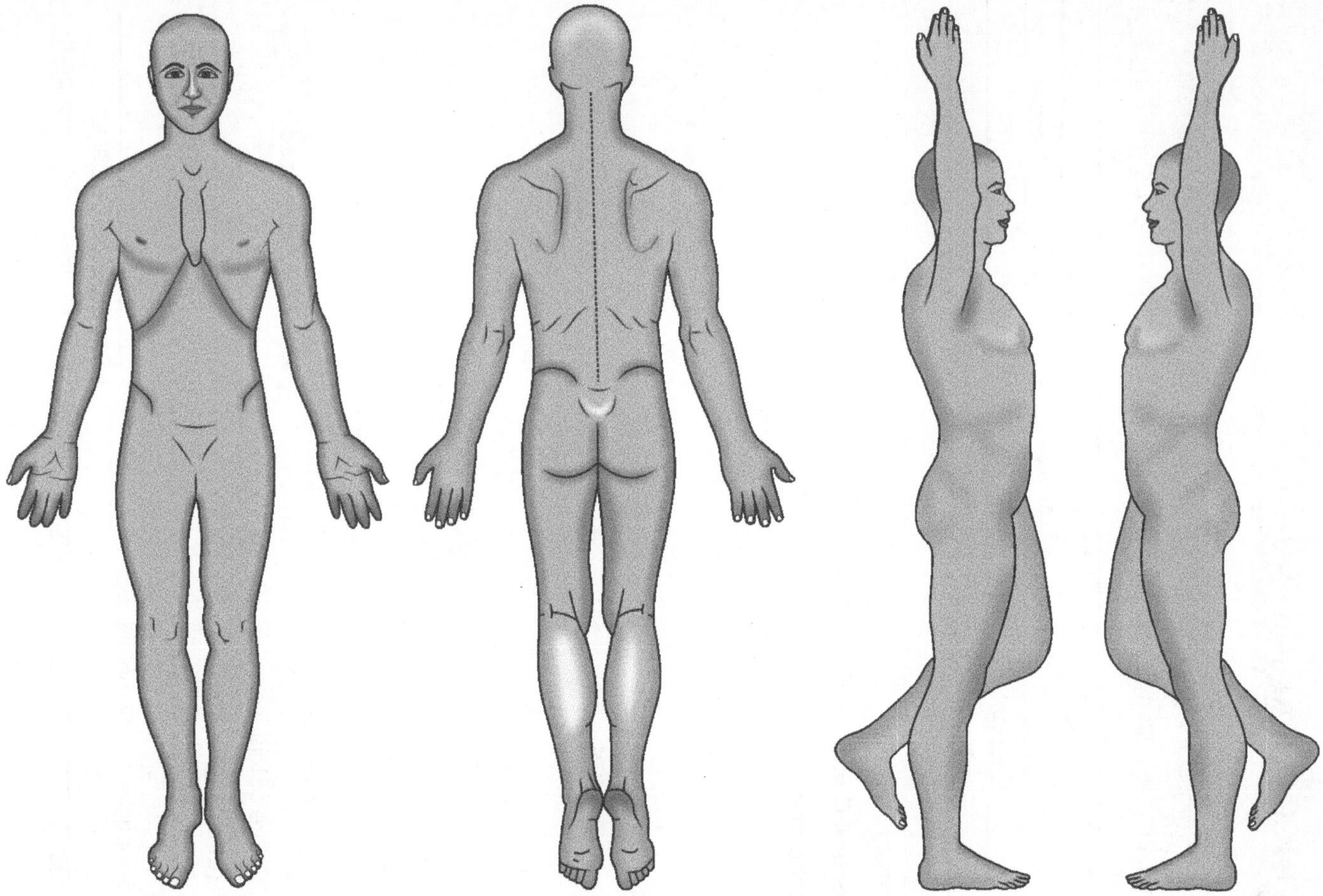

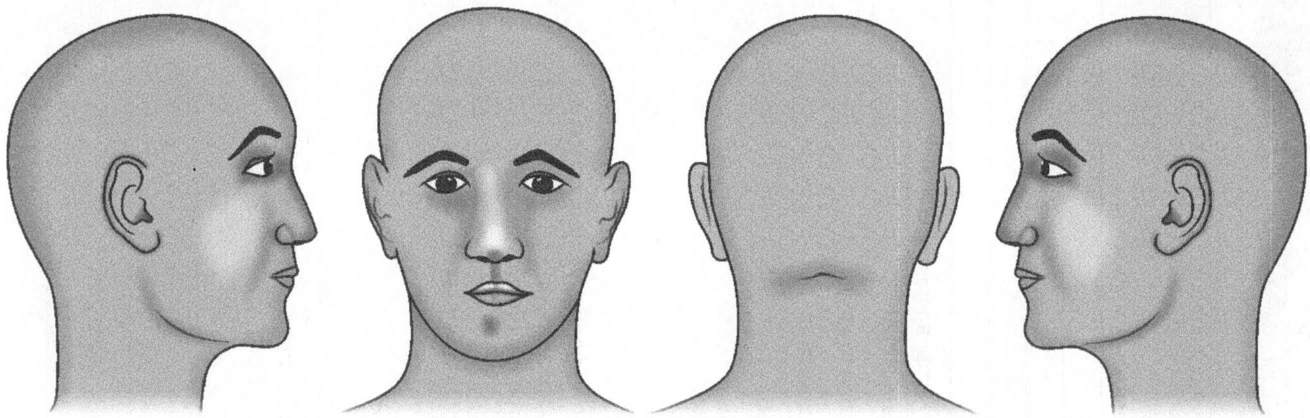

Signature of the Doctor
Name, Designation and Seal

EX. 4.5: MEDICOLEGAL REPORT II

Meera Devi, a 26-year-old female sustained second to third degree burns to her face and chest, entire left arm, anterior portion of her right arm and upper one-third of her abdomen when her in-laws and husband tried to burn her for dowry. She was rushed to the hospital by her neighbors. Remnants of burnt clothes were present on her body. Prepare a medicolegal report describing the burn injury.

CR. No. ____________ MLR No. ____________

Name ____________ S/ D/ W of ____________ Age ______ Gender ______

Residence ____________ Occupation ____________ Police Station ____________

Brought by ____________ Date and Time of Examination ____________

(If relative/ friend — Name, address and signature)

Date and time of admission ____________

No. and date of police docket ____________

No. and name of constable ____________

Articles handed over to the police

CONSENT

I am willing for my medicolegal examination.
I have not been examined earlier.
I will show all my injuries on my person.
I have been explained that the result of the examination may go in my favor or against me.

Signature/ Thumb Impression of patient/ guardian

History

General Condition (Vitals)

Particulars of Injuries

Identification Marks

1. ____________
2. ____________

1. Nature of Injuries ____________
   (Simple/ grievous)
   ____
2. Probable duration of injuries ____________
   ____

Kind of weapon used

____
Signature of the Doctor
Name, Designation and Seal

Date __________ **MLR No.** __________ **CR No.** __________

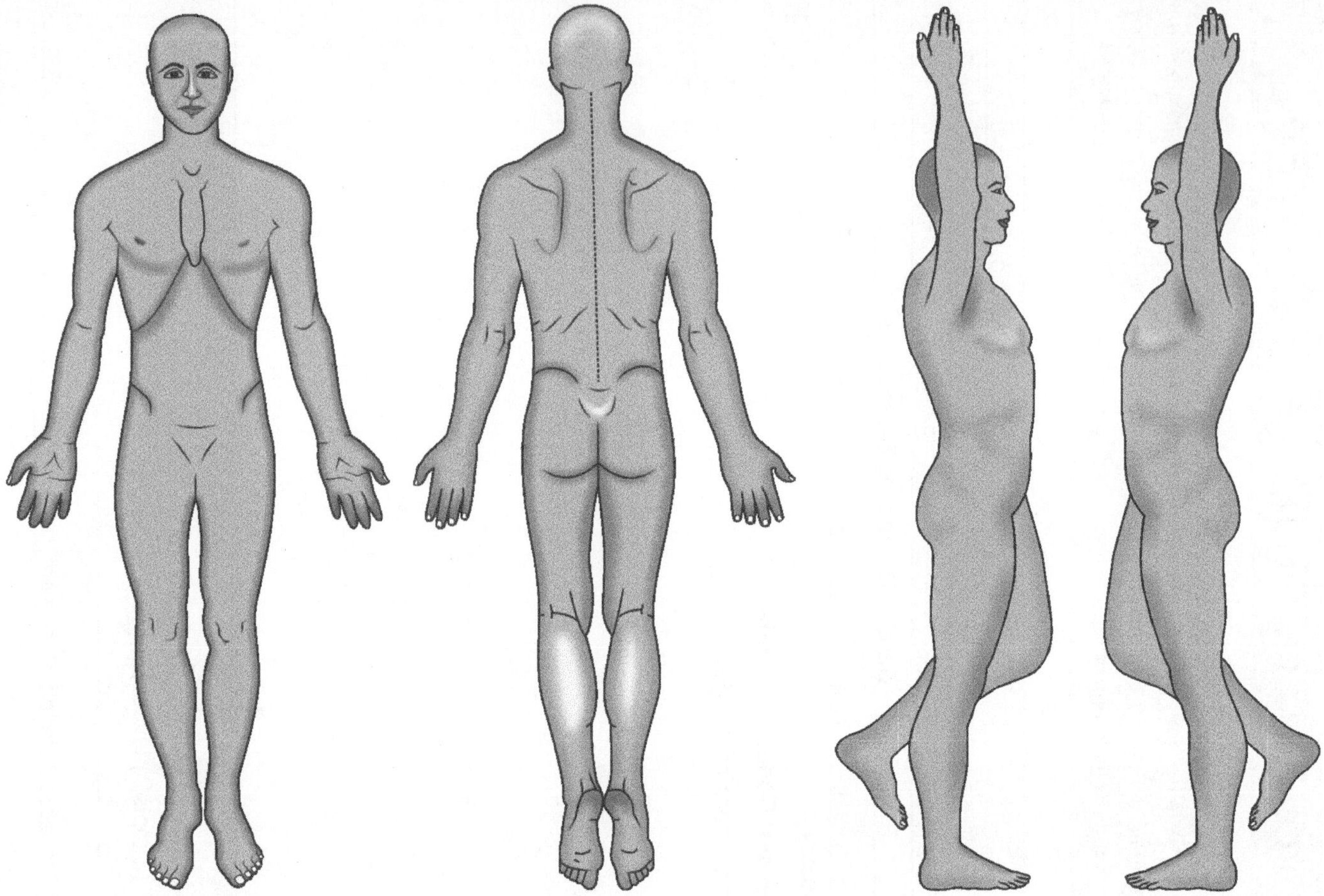

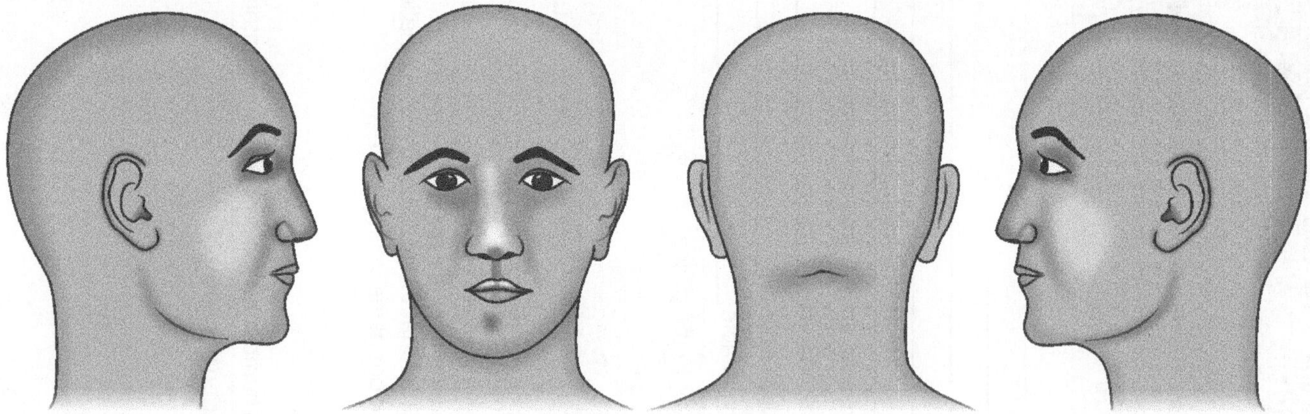

____

Signature of the Doctor
Name, Designation and Seal

EX. 4.6: MEDICOLEGAL REPORT III

A 36-year-old married female was allegedly assaulted by an unknown person with a knife when he tried to snatch her purse. She was brought to the casualty department with an elliptical stab wound on the left side of her chest and an incised wound on the left arm. Her vitals were B.P. 102/70 mm Hg, pulse: 92/min, respiratory rate: 22/min, and GCS: 15/15. She was wearing salwar kameez, bra and panty. Prepare a medicolegal report for the same.

CR. No. ______________ MLR No. ______________

Name ______________ S/ D/ W of ______________ Age ______ Gender ______

Residence ______________ Occupation ______________ Police Station ______________

Brought by ______________ Date and Time of Examination ______________

(If relative/ friend — Name, address and signature)

Date and time of admission ______________

No. and date of police docket ______________

No. and name of constable ______________

Articles handed over to the police

CONSENT

I am willing for my medicolegal examination.
I have not been examined earlier.
I will show all my injuries on my person.
I have been explained that the result of the examination may go in my favor or against me.

Signature/ Thumb Impression of patient/ guardian

History

General Condition (Vitals)

Particulars of Injuries

Identification Marks

1. ______________
2. ______________

1. Nature of Injuries ______________
   (Simple/ grievous)
   ____
2. Probable duration of injuries ______________
   ____

Kind of weapon used

____
Signature of the Doctor
Name, Designation and Seal

Date __________ **MLR No.** __________ **CR No.** __________

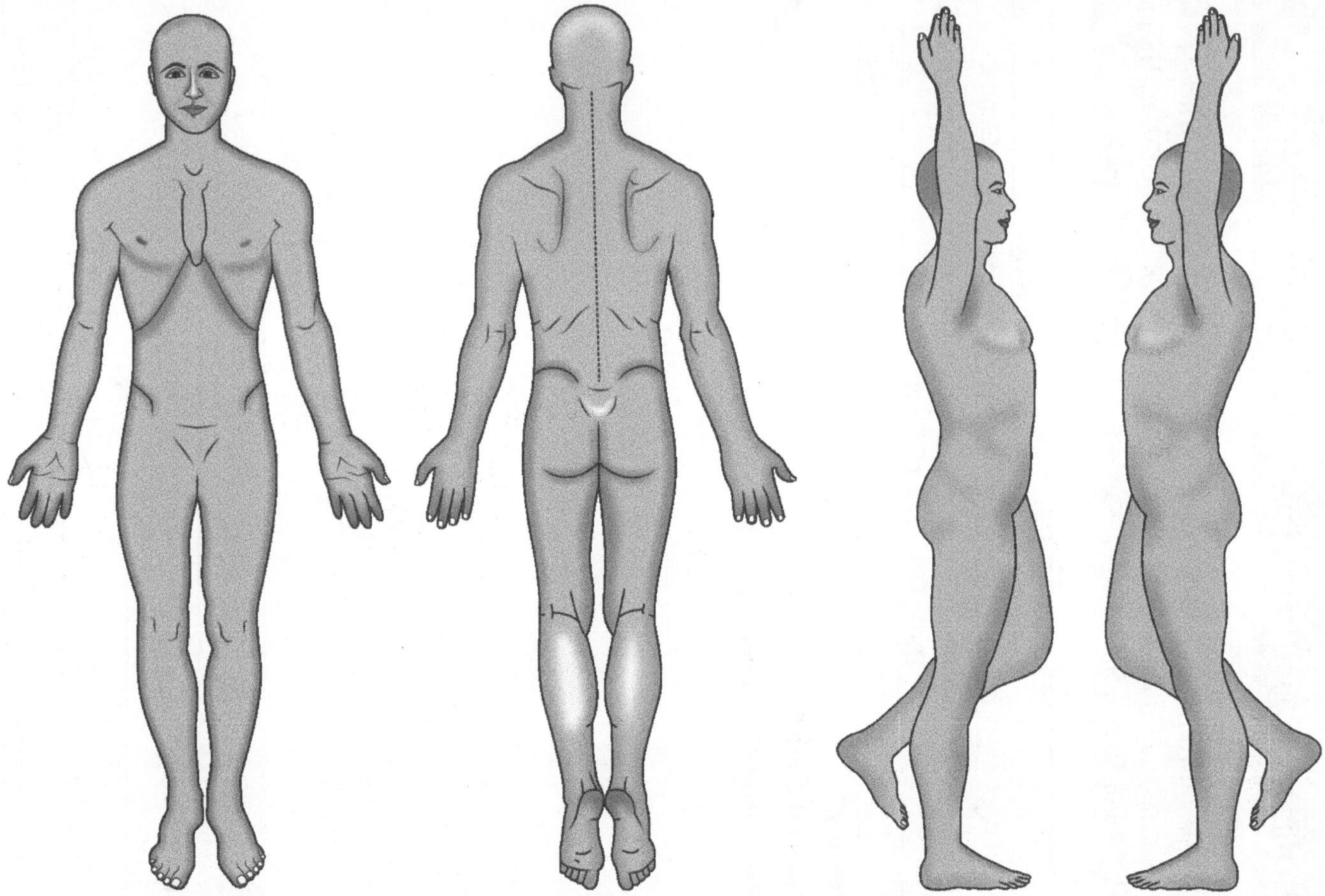

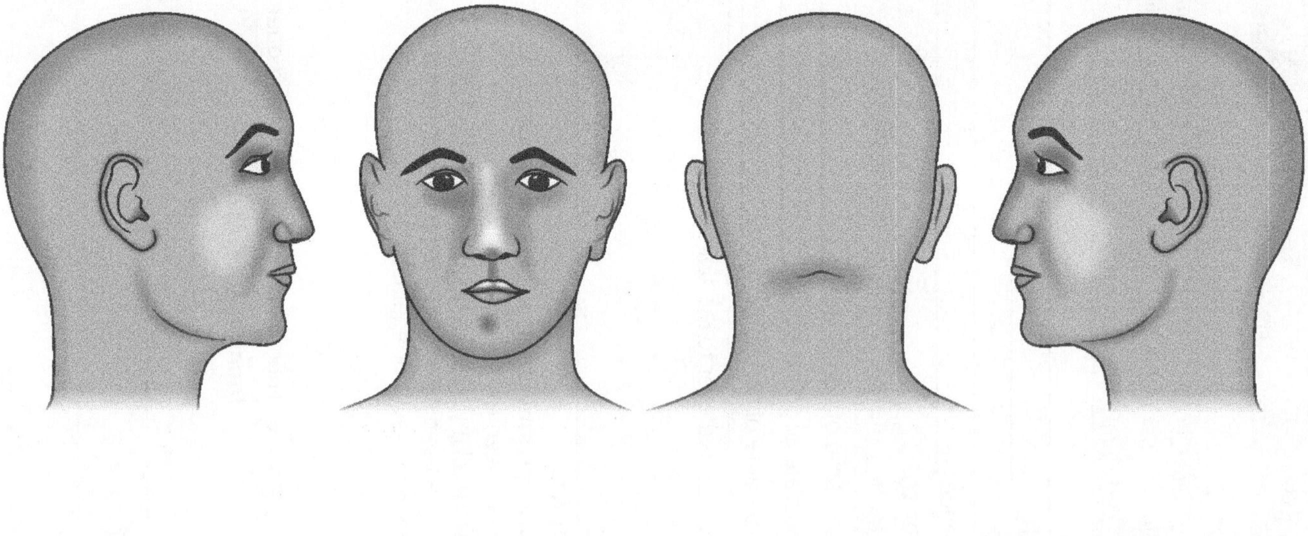

____

Signature of the Doctor
Name, Designation and Seal

EX. 4.7: MEDICOLEGAL REPORT IV

Dr Mani Venkataraman, a 56 year-old doctor suffered multiple gunshot injuries from an assault by an unknown person at about 5.30–5.45 AM while on his morning walk, when the person approached him and started shooting indiscriminately from a close range. He was immediately rushed to the hospital. There was one entry wound on right lateral chest wall in mid-axillary line and two entry and two exit bullet wounds on the right upper arm. He was wearing a track suit, vest and briefs at the time of incident. Prepare a medicolegal report for the same.

CR. No. ______ MLR No. ______

Name ______ S/ D/ W of ______ Age ______ Gender ______

Residence ______ Occupation ______ Police Station ______

Brought by ______ Date and Time of Examination ______

(If relative/ friend — Name, address and signature)

Date and time of admission ______

No. and date of police docket ______

No. and name of constable ______

Articles handed over to the police

CONSENT

I am willing for my medicolegal examination.
I have not been examined earlier.
I will show all my injuries on my person.
I have been explained that the result of the examination may go in my favor or against me.

Signature/ Thumb Impression of patient/ guardian

History

General Condition (Vitals)

Particulars of Injuries

Identification Marks

1. ______
2. ______

1. Nature of Injuries ______
(Simple/ grievous)
______

2. Probable duration of injuries ______
______

Kind of weapon used

______
Signature of the Doctor
Name, Designation and Seal

Date __________ MLR No. __________ CR No. __________

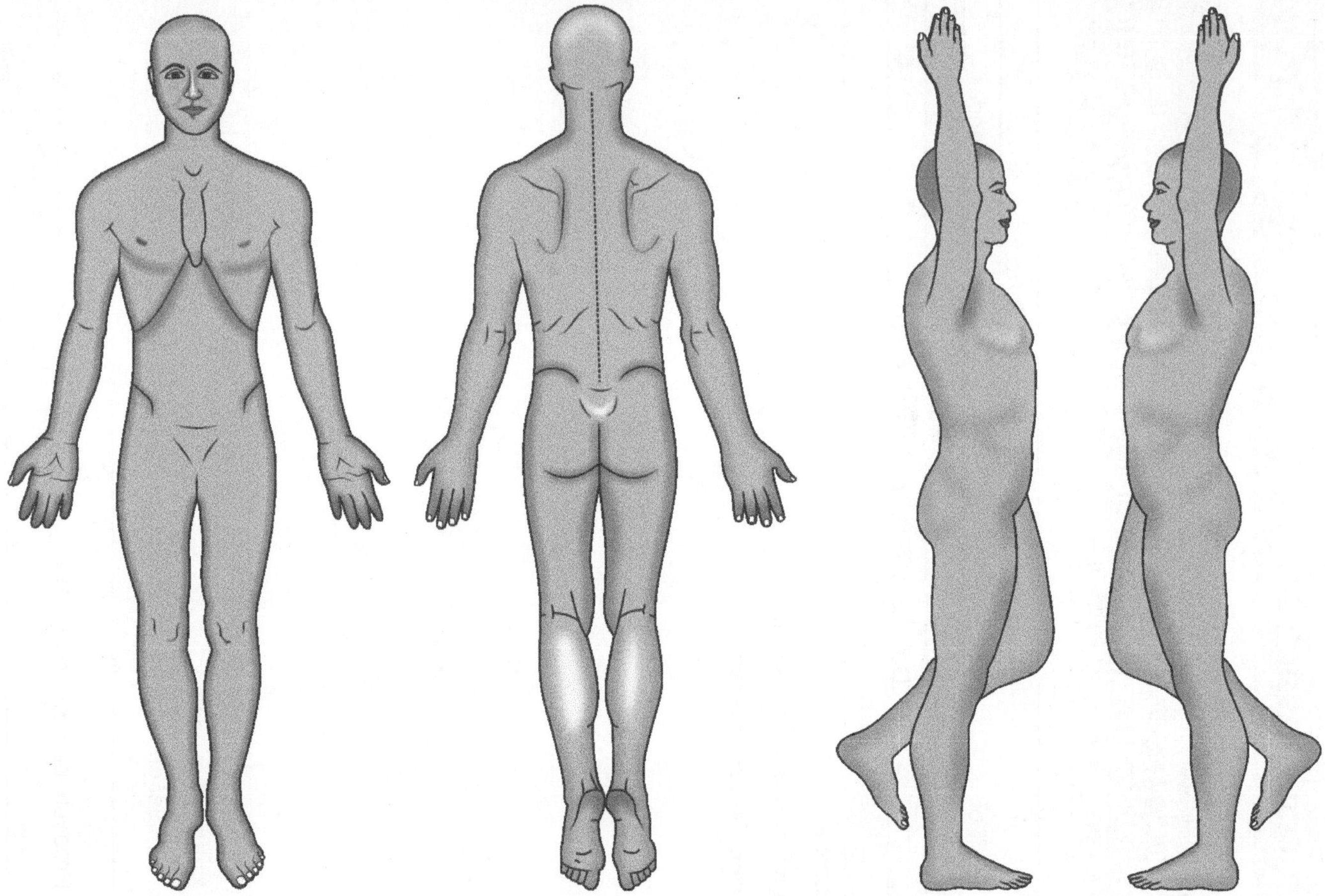

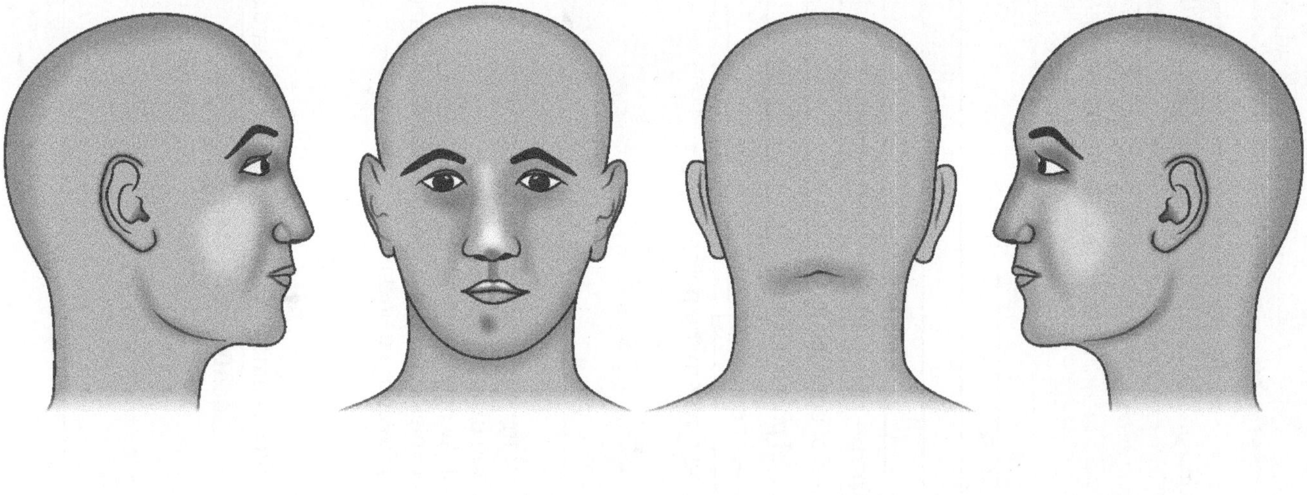

____
Signature of the Doctor
Name, Designation and Seal

EX. 4.8: MEDICOLEGAL REPORT V

CR. No. ________ MLR No. ________

Name ________ S/ D/ W of ________ Age ____ Gender ____

Residence ________ Occupation ________ Police Station ________

Brought by ________ Date and Time of Examination ________

(If relative/ friend — Name, address and signature)

Date and time of admission ________

No. and date of police docket ________

No. and name of constable ________

Articles handed over to the police

CONSENT

I am willing for my medicolegal examination.
I have not been examined earlier.
I will show all my injuries on my person.
I have been explained that the result of the examination may go in my favor or against me.

Signature/ Thumb Impression of patient/ guardian

History

General Condition (Vitals)

Particulars of Injuries

Identification Marks

1. ________
2. ________

1. Nature of Injuries ________
   (Simple/ grievous)
   ____
2. Probable duration of injuries ________
   ____

Kind of weapon used

____

Signature of the Doctor
Name, Designation and Seal

Date __________ MLR No. __________ CR No. __________

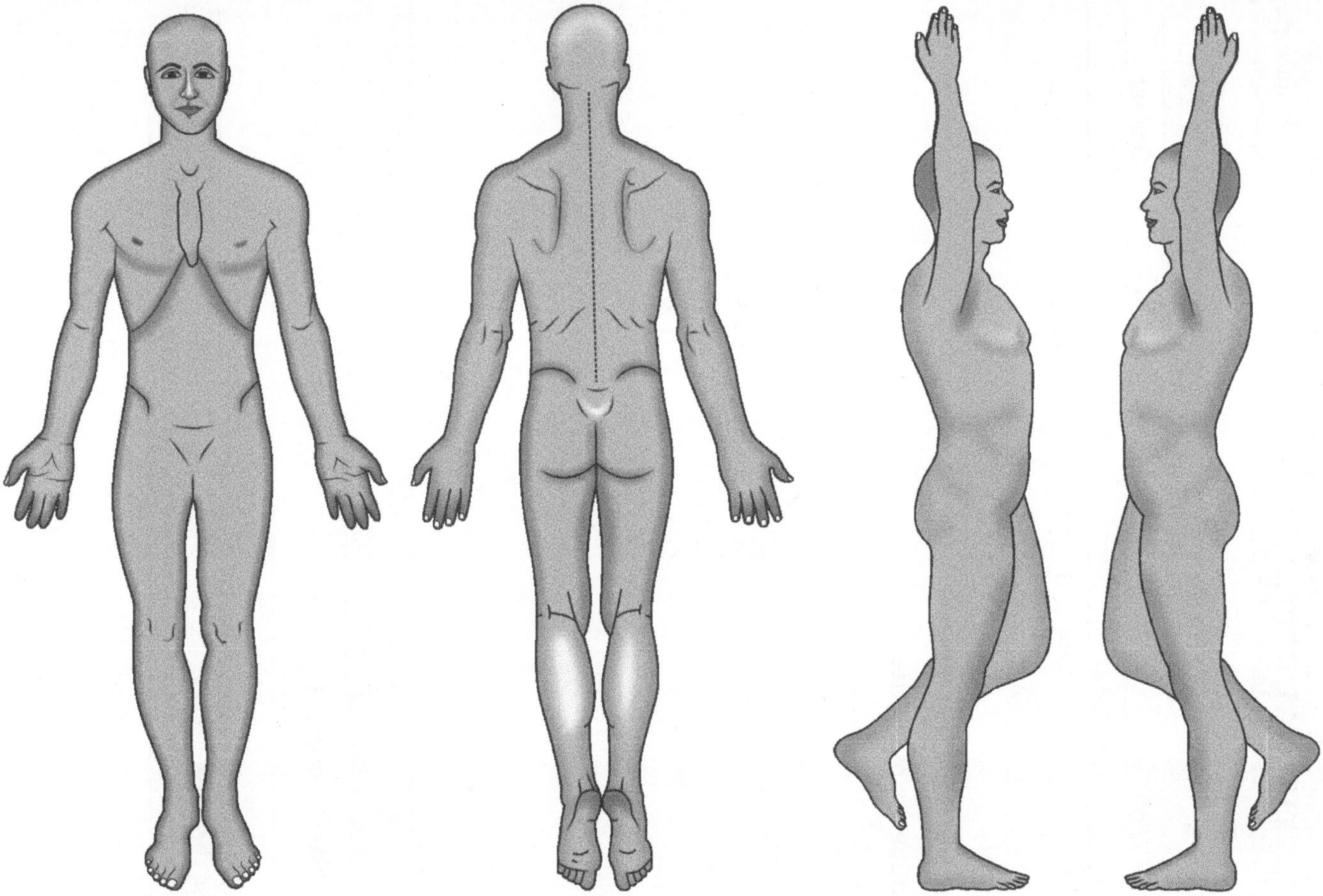

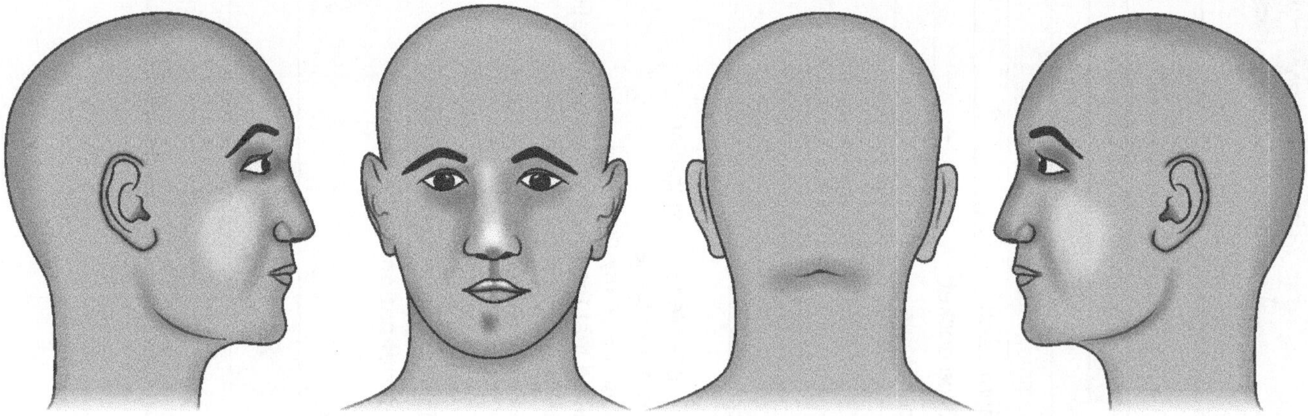

____
Signature of the Doctor
Name, Designation and Seal

EX. 4.9: REQUISITION FORM FOR INVESTIGATIONS

Department of Forensic Medicine and Toxicology

____

To Date __________

The Professor/ Medical Officer I/ C

Department of Radiology/ Pathology/ Biochemistry

____

Subject: X ray/ CT/ USG/ MRI scan/ Laboratory investigation required

Dear Sir/ Madam,

Ref.: MLC No. ______________ CR No. ______________ Dated ______________

I request that radiograph/ CT/ USG/ MRI/ ______________________ (investigations) of the subject

Mr/ Ms ________________ aged ______ years, resident of ________________

may be taken/ carried out as indicated below:

1. ______________________________
2. ______________________________
3. ______________________________

Brief history: ____

____

____

The subject bears the following identification marks:

1. ______________________________
2. ______________________________

I request you that the report and opinion may be sent to the undersigned at the earliest.

Thanking you

With regards,

____

Place __________ Signature of the Doctor

Name, Designation and Seal

Date __________

EX. 4.10: SUPPLEMENTARY REPORT

Department of Forensic Medicine and Toxicology

____

To Date ________________

The Investigating Officer,

______________________ Police Station,

________________District/ City/ Town

Subject: Supplementary report in case of Mr/ Ms ______________________________

S/ D/ W of ____________________________ vide MLR No. ________________________ dated __________________

Sir,

Keeping in view the ________________________ report nos. ______________________, I am of the opinion that injury nos. ____________________ are simple in nature, and injury nos. ________________ are grievous in nature.

With regards,

____

Signature of the doctor
Name, Designation and Seal

Enclosed: *(Tick '√')*

- ☐ __________ X-rays along with report in original duly initialed by me
- ☐ __________ CT along with report in original duly initialed by me
- ☐ Surgeon's report in original duly initialed by me
- ☐ Pathology report in original duly initialed by me

Received supplementary report along with _________________ X-rays and/ or ____________________ report (s).

Name _____________________________________ P.C. No. _________________________ P.S. _______________

____

Signature and date

EX. 4.11: EXAMINATION REPORT OF A WEAPON

Department of Forensic Medicine and Toxicology

____

To

The Investigation Officer,

__________ (Police Station)

__________ (Place)

Subject: Examination of the weapon provided (Reference letter No. __________

Dated __________)

Sir/ Madam

In reference to the above letter, I am sending you the report about the weapon sent in a parcel with __________ seals in connection with the injuries sustained by Mr/ Ms __________ S/ D/ W of __________ aged about __________ years (vide MLR No. __________ dated __________).

Description of the Weapon

(The weapon should preferably be examined after fingerprint and serological examination)

Name of weapon __________ Type of weapon __________

Shape (refer to the diagram) __________

Weapon (intact/ broken) __________

Weight __________
(in case of heavy blunt object)

Length __________ Width/ Circumference __________

Thickness/ diameter __________

Edges (margins)/ surface __________

Tip/ end __________

Handle __________

Joint __________ Type __________

Hilt __________

Trace evidence (hair/ fibers/ cloth/ stains/ rust), if any __________

Injuries possible __________

Identification marks, if any, on the weapon __________

Labeled Diagram

(Put signature and date with indelible ink on the weapon)

Opinion (*may be framed from any of the given sentences*)

- After examination of the weapon, I am of the opinion that injury No(s) ________, ________, ________, ________, is/ are possible with the given weapon.
- After examination of the weapon, I am of the opinion that injury No(s) ________, ________, ________, ________, is/ are not possible with the given weapon.
- After examination of the weapon, I am of the opinion that none/ all of the injuries mentioned are possible/ are not possible with the given weapon.

____

Place ______________ Signature of the Doctor

Date ______________ Name, Designation and Seal

Received report along with the weapon packed and sealed with ___________ seals.

Name ________________________________ P.C. No. ____________________ P.S. ________________

____

Signature and date

EX. 4.12: MEDICOLEGAL REPORT IN CASE OF POISONING

Manju Deshwal, a 21-year-old female, was brought to the emergency in unconscious state, with alleged history of ingestion of 20-25 tablets of benzodiazepines tablets 3 hours back. Off late, she was under stress, and tried to commit suicide because of breach of promise to marry by her partner. On examination, her GCS was 3, mild cyanosis and pallor was present. Pulse: 100/ min feeble, B.P. 82/ mm Hg systolic, respiratory rate 28/ min regular, Temperature - 36.4 °C. CNS examination showed deep coma, bilateral constricted pupils, which reacted minimally to light; diminished tendon reflexes and plantar reflexes were not elicitable bilaterally with retention of urine. There was no response to painful stimuli. Prepare a medicolegal report for the same.

Department of Forensic Medicine and Toxicology

____

MLR No. ____________ Date and time of examination ____________

Name ______________________ S/D/W of ______________________

Age ________ years Gender ____________

Address ______________________________

Brought by ______________________ Relation ____________

Consent I am willing for my medicolegal examination. I have not been examined earlier. I have been explained that the result of the examination may go in my favor or against. Signature/Thumb Impression of the person/ guardian	**Marks of Identification** 1. ______________________ ______________________ 2. ______________________ ______________________

Brief history the case: (Name of the person giving history ______________________)

(including symptoms, quantity, route, manner of exposure, date and time of onset)

____

____

____

____

Findings of Medical Examination

Clothings ______________________________

Pulse ______/ min B.P. ________ mm Hg Respiratory rate _____/ min

Temperature _____°C GCS ____________

Consciousness	☐ Fully conscious	☐ Drowsy	☐ Unconscious
Orientation (time, place, person)	☐ Well oriented	☐ Disoriented	
Memory (recent/ remote)	☐ Intact	☐ Impaired	
Mental status	☐ Normal ☐ Delirious	☐ Depressed ☐ Seizures (generalized/ partial)	☐ Agitated
Condition of skin	☐ Flushed ☐ Rash ☐ Discolored ____________	☐ Pale ☐ Blisters	☐ Dry ☐ Perspiration
Needle marks/ bite marks	☐ Absent	☐ Present (describe) ____________	
Eyes (conjunctivae)	☐ Normal	☐ Congested	
Pupils	☐ Normal	☐ Dilated	☐ Constricted
Mouth/ lips/ tongue	☐ Normal ☐ Bitten	☐ Moist ☐ Discolored	☐ Dry
Smell from expired breath	☐ Absent ☐ Present (garlicky/ kerosene-like/ fruity/ rotten eggs/ phenolic/ burnt rope/ bitter almonds/ ____________)		
Vomitus (note color, odor, amount)			
Urine/ stool (note color, consistency)			

(Tick '✓')

Systemic Examination

Central Nervous System ____________

Reflexes ____________

Chest ____________

Abdomen ____________

Material Preserved: Blood/ urine/ vomitus/ stool/ clothes/ suicidal note (if found)
(Tick '√')

Advice ____________

Opinion is reserved till receipt of chemical examiner's report with regards to kind of poison.

____

Place ____________ Signature of the Doctor

Date ____________ Name, Designation and Seal

EX. 4.13: EXAMINATION OF A CASE OF DRUNKENNESS

Truck driver Sarma Chaudhary, a 48-year-old male was allegedly involved in a road side accident wherein he crushed two laborers under the wheels of his truck who were sleeping on the pavement. Upon arrival at the accident scene at 2 AM, the police officer found him shouting meaninglessly and detected an alcoholic odor from his breath, bloodshot eyes and slurred speech. An inspection of his truck revealed 2 empty whiskey bottles. He stated that he had consumed '2 or 3 pegs' two to three hours prior to the accident. He was arrested for driving under the influence of alcohol (Sec. 185 Motor Vehicle Act) and Sec. 304A IPC, and brought for medicolegal examination. Prepare a report for the same.

Department of Forensic Medicine and Toxicology

____

MLR No. ____________ C.R. No. ____________

Patient Details

Name ______________________ S/ D/ W of ______________________

Address ____

Gender ____________ Age (as reported) ________ years

Educational status ____________ Occupation ____________

Examination Details

Date and time of examination ______________ Time of completion ______________

Requisition from ____________ Vide letter no. ________ Dated ____________

Brought by (Name and signature) ______________ P.C. No. ________ P.S. ________

Accompanied by (name and relation) ______________________________

Informed Consent

I, ______________________ S/ D/ W of ______________________ hereby agree for a complete physical examination, recording of findings, collection of specimens as necessary for laboratory analysis and any other investigations as recommended by the examining doctor and release of a report to the police officials/ court of law concerned. This procedure has been fully explained to me. Further, I have been explained that the result may go against me. This information may be used for teaching and research purposes provided no identifying data is released.

The above has been explained to me in ______________ language and I have fully understood the same and I am signing this consent by my own free will.

______________ ______________

Signature and name of the witness

Address ____________

Signature/ Thumb impression of patient/ guardian

Marks of Identification

1. ______________________________

2. ______________________________

Brief history of the case ______________________________

____

Narrated by ______________________________

Medical History

Current medical problems ______________________________

Past medical history ______________________________

Hearing problems ______________________________

Visual problems ______________________________ Use of spectacles/ Contact lens: Yes/ No

Balance problems ______________________________

Diabetes: Yes/ No If taking insulin, when and how much taken ______________

Epilepsy: Yes/ No Renal impairment: Yes/ No Hepatic impairment: Yes/ No

Prescribed medication ______________________________

Specific History of Alcohol Intake

Quantity of alcohol consumed in last 24 hours ______________ Type of liquor ______________

First drink at ______________ AM/ PM Last drink at ______________ AM/ PM

Last meal ______________ AM/ PM Type of meal ______________

Weekly alcohol intake ______________________________

Drug/ addiction ______________________________

Past psychiatric history ______________________________

Past self-harm attempts ______________________________

Previous trauma (particularly to head and extremities) ______________________________

Social history ______________________________

Family history ______________________________

General Physical Examination

Built: Well/ Average/ Poor Height _______ cm Weight _______ kg

Pulse _______/ min BP _________ mm Hg Respiratory rate _______/ min

Areas of the body examined *(note injuries on separate body diagrams)* ___________________________

____

Clothing	☐ Decent	☐ Soiled	☐ Torn	☐ Disordered
Demeanor/ behavior	☐ Sober ☐ Aggressive	☐ Abusive ☐ Boastful	☐ Talkative ☐ Calm	
Face	☐ Normal	☐ Flushed	☐ Pale	
Eyes				
Conjunctiva	☐ Normal	☐ Congested		
Pupils	☐ Normal	☐ Dilated	☐ Contracted	
Reaction to light	☐ Normal	☐ Delayed	☐ Sluggishly reacting	☐ Non-reacting
Visual acuity	☐ Normal	☐ Abnormal		
Nystagmus				
Horizontal gaze	☐ Coarse	☐ Fine	☐ Continuous	☐ Absent
Vertical gaze	☐ Yes	☐ No		
Convergence	☐ Yes	☐ No		
Ear (discharge)	☐ Yes	☐ No		
Mouth (signs of vomiting, salivation)	☐ Yes	☐ No		
Smell of alcohol	☐ Strong	☐ Moderate	☐ Faint	☐ None
Tongue	☐ Dry	☐ Moist	☐ Clean	☐ Furred
Speech	☐ Normal ☐ Overprecise	☐ Incoherent ☐ Thick and slurred	☐ Stuttering	
Gait	☐ Normal	☐ Broad-gauge	☐ Stumbling	☐ Self-control
Reflexes	☐ Normal	☐ Exaggerated	☐ Depressed (sluggish)	
Mental state				
Self-control	☐ Normal	☐ Impaired		
Memory	☐ Clear	☐ Vague	☐ Confused	
Orientation				
Time	☐ Good	☐ Moderate	☐ Bad	☐ Indefinite
Place	☐ Good	☐ Moderate	☐ Bad	☐ Indefinite
Reaction time	☐ Normal	☐ Delayed	☐ Increased	
Drug abuse	☐ Needle marks ☐ Rhinorrhea	☐ Shivering ☐ Gooseflesh	☐ Yawning ☐ Lachrymation	

(Tick '✓')

Specimen of handwriting ______________________________

Impairment Tests *(to determine incoordination)*

1. Romberg's Test				
Able to stand still during instructions	☐ Yes	☐ No		
Body swaying	☐ Marked	☐ Moderate	☐ Minimal	☐ Absent
Able to complete the test	☐ Yes	☐ No		
2. Walk and Turn Test				
Able to stand still during instructions	☐ Yes	☐ No		
Start too soon	☐ Yes	☐ No		
Stops walking	☐ Yes	☐ No		
Misses heel/ toe	☐ Yes	☐ No		
Gait on turning	☐ Normal	☐ Unsteady	☐ Stumbling	
Steps off line	☐ Yes	☐ No		
3. One Leg Stand Test				
Body swaying	☐ Marked	☐ Moderate	☐ Minimal	☐ Absent
Puts foot down	☐ Yes	☐ No		
Hops	☐ Yes	☐ No		
4. Finger and Nose Test				
Body swaying	☐ Marked	☐ Moderate	☐ Minimal	☐ Absent
Correct hand use	☐ Yes	☐ No		
Hand movements (incoordination)	☐ Marked	☐ Moderate	☐ Minimal	☐ Absent

(Tick '✓')

Systemic Examination

Cardiovascular System (heart sounds) ______________________________

Respiratory System (PN, breath sounds, added sounds) ______________________________

GIT Examination (Soft/ Tender/ Liver, Spleen, Kidneys/ Bowel sounds) ______________________________

____

Blood alcohol level (using breathalyzer or biochemical examination) ____________ mg%.

Sample preserved: Blood (in sodium fluoride and potassium oxalate) and urine (sodium fluoride) for FSL examination.

Opinion

Based on clinical and chemical examination, I am of the opinion that the above person has:

☐ Consumed alcohol and is under the influence of it.

☐ Consumed alcohol but is not under its influence.

☐ Not consumed alcohol.

(Tick '✓')

Place ___________ Signature of the Doctor

Date ___________ Name, Designation and Seal

Received MLR No. ______________________ along with a sealed glass vial, sample seal and an envelope addressed to chemical examiner.

Name ________________ P.C. No. ______________ P.S. ______________

Signature and date

EX. 4.14: PSYCHIATRIC ASSESSMENT OF A PERSON

Prabhu Iyengar a 22-year-old college student has been charged with murder after four students were stabbed to death at a party that was being held to celebrate the birthday of one of the victims. The accused was an invited guest to the party. He was arrested by the police, several buildings away from the site of murders. The knife used in the attack was also found in a nearby bush. The court has ordered for an assessment to determine whether he is mentally fit to stand trial. Prepare a report regarding the same.

Department of Forensic Psychiatry

____

MLR No. ________________ C.R. No. ________________

Patient Details

Name ______________________ S/ D/ W of ______________________

Address ______________________ Gender ______________________

Age (as reported) __________ years Date of birth (if known) ______________

Marital status: Unmarried/ Married/ Divorced Occupation ______________

Financial situation ______________ Educational status ______________

Examination Details

Date and time of examination ______________________ Time of completion ______________

Requisition from ______________ Vide letter no. ______________ Dated ______________

Brought by (Name and signature) ______________ P.C. No. ______________ P.S. ______________

Accompanied by (Name and relation) ______________________

Informed Consent

I, ______________________ S/ D/ W of ______________________ hereby agree for a complete physical examination, recording of findings, collection of specimens as necessary for laboratory analysis and any other investigations as recommended by the examining doctor and release of a report to the police officials/ court of law concerned. This procedure has been fully explained to me. Further, I have been explained that the result may go against me. This information may be used for teaching and research purposes provided no identifying data is released.

The above has been explained to me in ______________________ language and I have fully understood the same and I am signing this consent by my own free will.

______________________ ______________________

Signature of the witness Signature/ Thumb impression of patient/ guardian

Name and address ______________________

Marks of Identification

1. ____________________

2. ____________________

Brief history of the case ____________________

____

____

Narrated by ____________________

Psychiatric and Medical History

Presenting problem (onset, precipitants, duration, course) ____________________

____

____

Past medical history ____________________

Past psychiatric history ____________________

Past self-harm attempts ____________________

Previous trauma (especially head injury with +/ - LOC) ____________________

Prescribed medication ____________________

Drug/ addiction ____________________

Alcohol intake and weekly alcohol intake ____________________

Allergies ____________________

Social Circumstances (housing, employment, financial, relationships, life events) ____________________

____

Family History (social, medical and psychiatric) ____________________

____

Personal/ Developmental History

a. Childhood (family structure, parents' occupation, relationship with parents, siblings, friends, abuse) ____________________

____

b. Adolescence and teen (friends, relationships, school, activities, sex, trouble, relationship with parents) ____________________

____

c. Adulthood (work, finances, education, relationships, family, goals for future) ____________________

____

Mental State Examination

A. General description

Self-care/ appearance, e.g. clothing, facial expression, habits ______

Behavior, e.g. disinhibited, withdrawn, aggressive ______

Motor, e.g. retardation, overactivity, Parkinsonian ______

Attitude towards examiner, e.g. cooperative, friendly, hostile, resentful ______

B. Mood and affect

Mood, e.g. depressed, anxious, elation, irritability, fluctuating ______

Affect ______

Appropriateness ______

Biological symptoms, e.g. sleep, appetite, energy ______

C. Speech

Rate and quantity, e.g. fast, slow, monosyllabic, slurred ______

D. Perceptual disturbances

Delusions ______

Hallucinations, e.g. auditory, visual, tactile, olfactory, gustatory ______

Process or form of thought, e.g. paranoid, flight of ideas, thought blocking, thought insertion ______

______

E. Cognition

Alertness and level of consciousness ______

Orientation (time and place)______

Memory, e.g. short/ long-term ______

Concentration and attention ______

Intellectual disability including capacity to read and write ______

Visuospatial ability ______

Abstract thinking ______

Fund of information and intelligence ______

F. Obsessive compulsive phenomenon ______

G. Judgment and insight ______

H. Reliability ______

I. Risk behaviors (suicidal or homicidal thoughts) ______

General Physical Examination

Built: Well/ Average/ Poor Height _______ cm Weight _______ kg

Pulse _______/ min BP __________ mm Hg Respiratory rate _____/ min

General appearance ____________________

Areas of the body examined *(note injuries on separate body diagrams)* ____________________

____

Speech (articulation) ____________________

Eyes ____________________

Mouth ____________________ Tongue ____________________

Breath ____________________ Skin and lips ____________________

Drug misuse: Needle marks/ Shivering/ Yawning/ Rhinorrhea/ Gooseflesh/ Lachrymation

Systemic Examination

Cardiovascular System (Heart sounds) ____________________

Respiratory System (PN, breath sounds, added sounds) ____________________

GIT Examination (Soft/ Tender/ Liver, spleen, kidneys/ Bowel sounds) ____________________

____

CNS Examination (Power, tone, reflexes, coordination, gait, Romberg's) ____________________

____

Sample preserved: Blood, urine (if required)

Opinion

After complete medical and psychiatric evaluation and laboratory examination, I am of the opinion that the person requires compulsory admission/ no admission in the hospital. He is fit/ not fit to stand trial.

Place __________ Signature of the Doctor

Date __________ Name, Designation and Seal

Received MLR No. ____________________ along with laboratory reports.

Name ____________________ P.C. No. ____________________ P.S. ____________

Signature and date

EX. 4.15: EXAMINATION FOR EVIDENCE OF RECENT DELIVERY

Mithlesh Sinha, a 38 year-old mother of four female children, was charged with feticide (infanticide) after the local residents found a baby girl half-buried in the nearby forest. The baby was one day old when she was found wrapped in a cloth and half buried under earth and gravel, and died of her injuries two days later in hospital. Police believe the baby was abandoned by her family or close relative. The police brought her for examination to find out evidence to sustain the charge of murder and abandonment. Prepare an examination report of the female.

Department of Forensic Medicine and Toxicology

____

MLR No. ________________ C.R. No. ________________

Patient Details

Name ______________________________ D/ W of ______________________________

Address ____ Gender ____________________

Age (as reported) __________ years Date of birth (if known) ____________

Marital status: Unmarried/ Married/ Divorced Occupation __________________

Examination Details

Date and time of examination ____________________________ Time of completion __________________

Requisition from ________________________ Vide letter no. ________________ Dated ____________

Brought by (Name and signature) ______________________ P.C. No. ______________ P.S. ____________

Accompanied by (Name and relation) ____

Informed Consent

I, __________________________ D/ W of __________________________ hereby agree for a complete physical examination (including examination of genital organs), recording of findings, collection of specimens as necessary for laboratory analysis, photographic documentation and any other investigations as recommended by the examining doctor and release of a report to the police officials/ court of law concerned. This procedure has been fully explained to me. Further, I have been explained that the result may go against me. This information may be used for teaching and research purposes provided no identifying data is released.

The above has been explained to me in __________________________________ language and I have fully understood the same and I am signing this consent by my own free will.

________________________ ________________________

Signature of the witness Signature/ Thumb impression of patient/ guardian

Name and address ____________________

Signature and name of female nurse/ attendant (in case of male doctor) ______________________________

Marks of Identification

1. ______________________________

2. ______________________________

Brief history of the case (use separate sheet, if necessary) ______________________________

____

____

____

Menstrual/ Obstetric History

Age of menarche ____________ years/ Not attained/ Menopause attained

Periods (e.g. frequency/ regularity/ LMP) ______________________________

Menstruation at the time of examination ☐ Yes ☐ No

Antenatal check-up ☐ Taken ☐ Not taken

Mode of delivery ____________ Episiotomy ________

General Examination

Built: Well/ Average/ Poor Height ______ cm Weight ______ kg

Pulse ______/ min BP ________ mm Hg Respiratory rate _____/ min

General appearance ______________________________

Conscious level ______________________________

Demeanor/ behavior ☐ Sober ☐ Excited ☐ Calm ☐ Depressed

Pallor ☐ Present ☐ Absent

Chloasma ☐ Present ☐ Absent

Jaundice ☐ Present ☐ Absent

Systemic Examination Findings

Respiratory System ______________________________

Cardiovascular System ______________________________

Central Nervous System ______________________________

Specific Examination

Breasts			
Size, shape and consistency	☐ Engorged and pendulous	☐ Hemispherical, small and firm	
Veins	☐ Prominent	☐ Not prominent	
Striae	☐ Present	☐ Absent	
Areola	☐ Dark and prominent	☐ Pink and non-prominent	
Montgomery's tubercles	☐ Prominent	☐ Not prominent	
Nipples			
Size	☐ Well formed	☐ Small	
Color	☐ Pigmented	☐ Pink	
Surface	☐ Cracked	☐ Normal	
Colostrum/ milk	☐ Can be expressed	☐ Cannot be expressed	
Abdomen			
Shape, surface	☐ Pendulous with wrinkled skin	☐ Non-pendulous with smooth skin	
Striae gravidarum	☐ Present If present, color: Reddish/ Healed scar	☐ Absent	
Linea nigra	☐ Present	☐ Absent	
Uterus	☐ Palpable per abdomen If palpable: Level of upper border ____________________	☐ Not palpable per abdomen	
Examination of Genitalia			
Vulval pad (if present)	☐ Wet Color: Reddish/ Yellowish/ Whitish	☐ Not wet	
Perineum	☐ Episiotomy incision/ scar	☐ Normal	
Labia	Swollen/ Not swollen Gaping/ Not gaping Tears ☐ Present	Congested/ Not congested Tender/ Nontender ☐ Absent	
Fourchette	☐ Fresh tear	☐ Healed scar	☐ Intact
Posterior commissure	☐ Fresh tear	☐ Healed scar	☐ Intact
Vagina	Color: Purple/ Red Capacity: Capacious and relaxed/ Narrow with normal tone PV: Admits one finger with/ without pain/ Admits two fingers with/ without pain	Rugae: Marked/ Less obvious	
Cervix	Cervical lips: Soft and swollen/ Firm Cervical mucus plug: Present/ Absent External Os: Closed/ Open Shape: Circular, dimple like/ Transverse slit PV: Admits one finger/ Admits two fingers Injuries: Present/ Absent Lochia at Os: Present/ Absent If present, describe ______________		
Uterus	_______ weeks/ Non-pregnant Adnexa ____________________	Tender/ Nontender	

Tick ('✓')

Laboratory examinations: Urine for pregnancy test: Positive/ Negative

USG Abdomen (Optional):____

Any other ____

OPINION

i. After general, local and laboratory examination, I am of the opinion that the findings are suggestive/ not suggestive of recent delivery.

ii. Approximate period elapsed since delivery is about __________________ days/ weeks/ months.*

*(*Strike out, if not applicable)*

____

Place ___________ Signature of the Doctor

Date___________ Name, Designation and Seal

Received MLR No.___________________

Name ______________________________ P.C. No. ______________________ P.S. __________________________

____

Signature and date

NOTES

NOTES

NOTES

UNIT V

Sexual Offences

EXAMINATION OF SURVIVOR

Survivor: The term 'survivor' is preferably used instead of 'victim' since it recognizes that the person is capable of taking decisions despite being victimized, humiliated and traumatized due to the assault.

It must be understood that forensic medical examination of the victim is a 'medicolegal emergency' as per the Supreme Court guidelines. Hence, such cases must be examined without delay. No such case should be refused for examination for the reasons of nonavailability of lady medical officer, because as per 164 A Criminal Procedure Code (CrPC), any registered medical practitioner can examine victim in presence of other woman with the consent of the patient or guardian.

Medical Examination of the Victim of Rape (Sec. 164A CrPC)

1. Where, during the stage when an offence of committing rape or attempt to commit rape is under investigation, it is proposed to get the woman with whom rape is alleged or attempted to have been committed or attempted, examined by a medical expert, such examination shall be conducted by a registered medical practitioner (RMP) employed in a hospital run by the Government or a local authority and in the absence of a such a practitioner, by any other registered medical practitioner, with the consent of such woman or of a person competent to give such consent on her behalf and such woman shall be sent to such RMP within 24 hours from the time of receiving the information relating to the commission of such offence.
2. The RMP, to whom such woman is sent shall, without delay, examine her and prepare a report of his/her examination giving the following particulars, namely:
   a. The name and address of the woman and of the person by whom she was brought;
   b. The age of the woman;
   c. The description of material taken from the person of the woman for DNA profiling;
   d. Marks of injury, if any, on the person of the woman;
   e. General mental condition of the woman; and
   f. Other material particulars in reasonable detail.
3. The report shall state precisely the reasons for each conclusion arrived at.
4. The report shall specifically record that the consent of the woman or of the person competent to give such consent on her behalf to such examination had been obtained.
5. The exact time of commencement and completion of the examination shall also be noted in the report.
6. The RMP shall, without delay forward the report to the investigation officer who shall forward it to the Magistrate referred to in Sec. 173 as part of the documents referred to in clause (a) of subsection (5) of that section.
7. Nothing in this section shall be construed as rendering lawful any examination without the consent of the woman or of any person competent to give such consent on her behalf.

Explanation: For the purposes of this section, 'examination' and 'registered medical practitioner' shall have the same meanings as in Sec. 53 CrPC.

'Two-finger test': The Supreme Court has described this test to determine the 'laxity' of vagina as *'unscientific, inhuman and degrading'*. It cannot be used against a woman, and that a rape survivor's 'habituation to sexual intercourse' is immaterial. The test is often used by defendant's lawyer to label victims as 'loose women', and identified as being 'habituated to sex'.

The samples must be collected as per time elapsed between assault and examination, history and physical findings. This will avoid unnecessary sample collection.

The *provisional opinion* must, in brief, mention relevant aspects of the history of sexual violence, clinical findings and samples which are sent for analysis to FSL. The report should contain negative as well as positive findings. An inference must be drawn in the opinion, correlating the history and clinical findings (Table 5.1). Absence of body/ genital injuries on victim of sexual assault does not rule out commission of the offence.

The *final opinion* of whether sexual intercourse has taken place or not is based on a consideration of (Table 5.1):

a. Signs of struggle.
b. Presence of blood and/ or seminal stains on clothes and body.
c. Presence of seminal matter in the vagina.
d. Transmission of venereal disease.
e. Forensic science laboratory reports

EXAMINATION OF ACCUSED

Examination of Accused by Medical Practitioner at the Request of Police Officer (Sec. 53 CrPC)

1. When a person is arrested on a charge of committing an offence of such a nature and alleged to have been committed under such circumstances that there are reasonable grounds for believing that an examination of his person will afford evidence as to the commission of an offence, it shall be lawful for a RMP, acting at the request of a police officer not below the rank of Sub-Inspector, and for any person acting in good faith in his aid and under his direction, to make such an examination of the person arrested as is reasonable necessary in order to ascertain the facts which may afford such evidence, and to use such force as is reasonably necessary for that purpose.
2. Whenever the person of a female is to be examined under this section, the examination shall be made only by, or under the supervision of, a female RMP.

Examination of Accused of Rape by Medical Practitioner (Sec. 53A CrPC)

1. When a person is arrested on a charge of committing an offence of rape or an attempt to commit rape and there are reasonable grounds for believing that an examination of his person will afford evidence as to the commission of such offence, it shall be lawful for a RMP employed in a hospital run by the Government or by a local authority and in the absence of such a practitioner within the radius of 16 kilometers from the place where the offence has been committed by any other RMP, acting at the request of a police officer not below the rank of a Sub-Inspector, and for any person acting in good faith in his aid and under his direction, to make such an examination of the arrested person and to use such force as is reasonably necessary for that purpose.
2. The RMP conducting such examination shall, without delay, examine such person and prepare a report of his/her examination giving the following particulars, namely:
   a. The name and address of the accused and of the person by whom he was brought
   b. The age of the accused, marks of injury, if any, on the person of the accused
   d. The description of material taken from the person of the accused for DNA profiling
   e. Other material particulars in reasonable detail.
3. The report shall state precisely the reasons for each conclusion arrived at.
4. The exact time of commencement and completion of the examination shall also be noted in the report.
5. The RMP shall, without delay, forward the report of the investigating officer, who shall forward it to the Magistrate referred to in Sec. 173 as part of the documents referred to in clause (a) of Subsection (5) of that section.

Table 5.1: Drafting of opinion based on examination findings and FSL report

Genital injuries	Physical injuries	Provisional opinion	FSL report	Final opinion
Present	Present	There are signs suggestive of recent forceful penetration of vagina/ anus. Opinion regarding intercourse is reserved till FSL report is received.	Positive for presence of semen	There are signs suggestive of recent forceful vaginal/ anal intercourse.
			Negative for presence of semen/ lubricant	There are no signs suggestive vaginal/ anal intercourse, but evidence of physical and genital assault present.
Present	Absent	There are signs suggestive of recent forceful penetration of vagina/ anus.	Positive for presence of semen	There are signs suggestive of recent forceful vaginal/ anal intercourse.
			Negative for presence of semen/ lubricant	There are no signs suggestive of recent vaginal/ anal intercourse, but there is evidence of genital assault.
Absent	Present	There are signs of use of force, however, final opinion is reserved pending availability of FSL reports.	Positive for semen	There are signs suggestive of forceful vaginal/ anal intercourse.
			Negative for semen/ lubricant	There are no signs suggestive of vaginal/ anal intercourse, but there is evidence of physical assault.
Absent	Absent	There are no signs of use of force; however final opinion is reserved pending availability of FSL reports.	Positive for semen	There are signs suggestive of vaginal/ anal intercourse.
			Positive for semen and alcohol	There are signs suggestive of vaginal/ anal intercourse under the influence of alcohol.
			Positive for lubricant	There is a possibility of vaginal/ anal penetration by lubricated object.
			Negative for semen/ alcohol/ lubricant	There are no signs suggestive of vaginal/ anal intercourse or penetration of vagina/ anus.

EX. 5.1: EXAMINATION OF SURVIVOR OF SEXUAL VIOLENCE

Chandrika Khobragade, a 16 year-old-girl was brought by the police with alleged history of rape by her neighbor. She was raped in the fields when she had gone there to attend nature's call. She is thin built, 154 cm tall and weighed 48 kg. The victim presented with torn garments at places, stained with mud and sand particles, and stated that she has been raped at knife-point. The incident happened between 8.00 to 9.00 PM and she was brought to the emergency by the constable for examination at 11 PM on the same day. Prepare a medicolegal report for the same.

Department of Forensic Medicine and Toxicology

____

MLR No. ________________ CR. No. ________________

Patient Details

Name ________________________________ D/ W/ S of ______________________

Address ____

Age (as reported) ________ years Date of birth (if known) ________________

Gender ________________ Marital status: Unmarried/ Married/ Divorced

Occupation ____________________________ Educational status ____________________________

Contact phone no. (if any) ________________________________

Examination Details

Date and Time of arrival in the hospital ____________________________

Date and Time of commencement of examination____________________________________

Brought by (Name and signatures)

a. If police: Name _____________________ P.C. No.________________ P.S.__________________________

b. If not brought by police, name and relation with the examinee ____________________________________

Any identified special needs/ mental health problems ____
(Interpreters or special educators will be needed where the survivor has special needs such as hearing/ speech disability, language barriers, intellectual or psychosocial disability)

Name of Social worker/ Care worker (if any) ____

Informed Consent

I, ____ D/ W/ S of ______________________________

hereby voluntary consent and agree to the following: *(Tick '√')*

☐ Medical examination for treatment

☐ Medicolegal examination

☐ Sample collection for clinical and forensic examination

I understand that the medicolegal examination will include:

- A full medical history and complete examination (including examination of genital organs);
- Collection of forensic and medical specimens;
- Taking of notes, photographs/ digital images for recording and evidential purposes;
- I understand and agree that a copy of the medical notes may be given to professionals involved in the case (e.g. police or lawyers) and may be used in the court;
- I agree to the use of my anonymized photographs/ digital images/ medical notes for teaching, audit and research;
- I have been informed that I may halt the examination at anytime with possible consequences of such refusal viz. loss of evidence and documentation. I have been further informed that this refusal will not effect my medical treatment.
- I also understand that as per law the hospital is required to inform police and this has been explained to me.

I want the information to be revealed to the police ☐ Yes ☐ No

The above have been explained to me in ______________________ language with the help of a special educator/ interpreter/ support person *(circle as appropriate)*.

Date____________

Name and signature (thumb impression) of survivor
(Parents/ guardian/ person in whom the child reposes trust in case of child < 12 years)

Signature and name of witness along with date and time ______________________________

Signature and name of special educator/ interpreter has ______________________________

Signature and name of female nurse/ attendant (in case of male doctor) ______________________

Marks of Identification

1. ____

2. ____

Brief history of assault (use separate sheet, if necessary) ______________________________

____

____

____

Narrator of the incident (specify name and relation to survivor, if not self) ______________________

Details of Assailant(s)

Number of assailants and name/ (s) ______________________________

Sex of assailant(s) ______________ Age of assailant(s) ______________

Prior knowledge of assailant(s) (relationship with the survivor) ______________________________

Last contact with alleged assailant(s) ______________________________

Medical History

General health ______________________________

Pre-existing skin problems, e.g. eczema, lichen sclerosus ______________________________

Previous illnesses ______________________________

Operations ______________________________

Menstrual/ Obstetric History

Age of menarche ________ years/ Not attained/ Menopause attained

Periods (e.g. frequency/ regularity/ LMP) ______________________________

Pre-existing menstrual problems, e.g. intermenstrual and postcoital bleeding ______________________________

Menstruation at the time of incident ☐ Yes ☐ No

Menstruation at the time of examination ☐ Yes ☐ No

Post assault, has there been any vaginal discharge/ bleeding? ☐ Yes ☐ No

Prior assault, has there been any vaginal discharge/ bleeding? ☐ Yes ☐ No

Was the survivor pregnant at time of incident? ☐ Yes ☐ No

If yes, duration of pregnancy ______________ weeks

Any children ______________ Mode of delivery ______________ Episiotomy ______________

Medications and Allergies

Prescribed medication ______________________________

Vaccination status: Tetanus (Vaccinated/ Not vaccinated)

Hepatitis B (Vaccinated/ Not vaccinated)

Allergies ______________________________

DETAILS OF THE ASSAULT FROM EXAMINEE

Specific Information Relating to the Alleged Offence

Date and Time of assault ________________ Time interval to examination ________________

Type of surface where assault occurred ________________

Whether sleeping or unconscious at the time of the incident? ________________

Whether cried for help or struggled or resisted? ________________

Query	Tick '√'	Details
Kissing/ licking/ biting/ sucking/ spitting *(sites)*	☐ Not Known ☐ No ☐ Yes	
Penile-oral penetration	☐ Not Known ☐ No ☐ Yes	
Digital penetration	☐ Not Known ☐ No ☐ Yes	
Penile-vaginal penetration	☐ Not Known ☐ No ☐ Yes	
Mouth to genitalia/ anus	☐ Not Known ☐ No ☐ Yes	
Penile-anal penetration	☐ Not Known ☐ No ☐ Yes	
Object to vulva/ vagina/ anus	☐ Not Known ☐ No ☐ Yes	
Other sexual/ physical act(s)	☐ Not Known ☐ No ☐ Yes	
Ejaculation onto skin/ hair	☐ Not Known ☐ No ☐ Yes	
Condom used throughout	☐ Not Known ☐ No ☐ Yes	
Lubricant/ spermicide used	☐ Not Known ☐ No ☐ Yes	
Injuries	☐ Not Known ☐ No ☐ Yes	
Anogenital bleeding	☐ Not Known ☐ No ☐ Yes	
Damage to clothing	☐ Not Known ☐ No ☐ Yes	

Threat Used During Assault

a. Physical violence (*Tick '√'*)

☐ Hit with hand, fist, blunt object, sharp object	☐ Bitten	☐ Pulled hair
☐ Burned	☐ Kicked	☐ Pinched
☐ Violently shaken	☐ Head banged	☐ Dragged

b. Emotional abuse (insulting, cursing, belittling, terrorizing) ________________

c. Use of restraints, if any ________________

d. Used or threatened the use of weapon(s) or objects, if any ________________

e. Verbal threats (e.g. threats of killing or hurting survivor or any other person in whom the survivor is interested; use of photographs for blackmailing, etc.), if any: ________________

f. Luring (sweets, chocolates, money or job), if any: ________________

g. Any other ________________

If survivor has left any marks of injury on assailant/ s (details) ________________

Aggravating factors, e.g. injuries in contact with assailant's blood or semen ☐ No ☐ Yes

Post Assault (*Ask if relevant*)

☐ Brushed teeth/ gums/ dentures ☐ Mouthwash/ spray used

☐ Washed/ bathed/ douched ☐ Changed tampon/ pad/ sponge/ diaphragm

Oral intercourse: Drank/ eaten food	☐ Not Known ☐ No ☐ Yes
Anal intercourse: Defecated since offence	☐ Not Known ☐ No ☐ Yes
Genital/ anal/ relevant skin: Wiped/ washed Specify site and disposal of cloth/ tissue	☐ Not Known ☐ No ☐ Yes _______________
Passed urine	☐ Not Known ☐ No ☐ Yes (note time)
Changed/ washed clothes If changed, are the clothes available?	☐ Not Known ☐ No ☐ Yes ☐ No ☐ Yes
Cleaned/ washed undergarments	☐ Not Known ☐ No ☐ Yes
Self-harm	(sites)

Direct Questions (*Ask if relevant*)

Complaint	Since assault	Details (If yes, note if this was previously experienced)
Abdominal pain		
Urinary symptoms (e.g. dysuria, frequency, hematuria, incontinence, UTI)		
Genital symptoms (e.g. soreness, discharge, bleeding, dysperunia, pruritis, injuries)		
Bowel symptoms (e.g. soreness, pain on defecation, discharge, bleeding, change in bowel habit, incontinence, pruritis, injuries)		

Sexual History

Dates and times of consensual sexual activity within the previous 10 days ____________________

Items used in previous intercourse

Condom ☐ Not Known ☐ No ☐ Yes

Spermicide ☐ Not Known ☐ No ☐ Yes

Lubricant ☐ Not Known ☐ No ☐ Yes

If relevant, clarify types of intercourse in last 10 days only: ____________________

Drug and Alcohol use in Relation to Assault

Was alcohol consumed? ☐ Not Known ☐ No ☐ Yes

If yes, please specify ☐ Post Offence ☐ Prior ☐ During

Start time of drinking ____________ End time of drinking ____________

Quantity and type of beverage consumed ____________

Time last ate ____________

Any illicit drugs been used/ administered to the survivor within 4 days of the examination? ☐ Not Known ☐ No ☐ Yes

If yes, please specify ☐ Post Offence ☐ Prior ☐ During

Give details ____________

Are any other substances having been used/ administered that could be relevant to the offence? ☐ Not Known ☐ No ☐ Yes

If yes, please specify ☐ Post Offence ☐ Prior ☐ During

Give details ____________

General Examination

Clothes

- Condition of clothes: Tears/ cuts/ rents/ burnt
- Foreign matter/ Stains: Blood/ seminal/ fecal/ mud/ grass/ any other ____________
- Buttons: Intact/ undone/ broken/ torn

Built: Well/ Average/ Poor

Height ______ cm Weight ______ kg

Pulse ______/ min BP ______ mm Hg Respiratory rate ______/ min

Conscious level ____________

General appearance ____________

Skin (color, gooseflesh, etc.) ____________

Hair (hair style, last wash, any added hair dye) ____________

Demeanor/ behavior ☐ Sober ☐ Eccentric ☐ Erratic ☐ Calm ☐ Depressed

Speech (e.g. content, form) ____________

Pre-existing physical problems (note type) ____________

Secondary sexual characters ____________

____

Injuries (Type, site, size, shape, color, swelling and signs of healing)

Site Examined		Injuries	Type of injury	Features/ Remarks
Scalp		☐ No ☐ Yes		
Face		☐ No ☐ Yes		
Eyes		☐ No ☐ Yes		
Ears		☐ No ☐ Yes		
Lips		☐ No ☐ Yes		
Inside mouth/ palate		☐ No ☐ Yes		
Teeth		☐ No ☐ Yes		
Neck		☐ No ☐ Yes		
Back		☐ No ☐ Yes		
Buttocks		☐ No ☐ Yes		
Arms	Right	☐ No ☐ Yes		
	Left	☐ No ☐ Yes		
Hands/ wrists	Right	☐ No ☐ Yes		
	Left	☐ No ☐ Yes		
Fingers/ nails	Right	☐ No ☐ Yes		
	Left	☐ No ☐ Yes		
Breasts		☐ No ☐ Yes		
Abdomen		☐ No ☐ Yes		
Legs	Right	☐ No ☐ Yes		
	Left	☐ No ☐ Yes		
Feet/ ankles/ soles	Right	☐ No ☐ Yes		
	Left	☐ No ☐ Yes		
Additional details (injection sites, self-harm, etc.)				

(Tick '✓')

Systemic Examination

Cardiorespiratory System

Heart sounds, Trachea/ air entry, breath sounds ____________________

____

Abdomen

Liver, Kidneys, Spleen ____________________

Tenderness/ masses ____________________

Bowel sounds ____________________

Central Nervous Systems

Pupil size and reactions ____________________

Eye movement/ nystagmus ____________________

Conjunctivae ____________________

Balance/ coordination ____________________

Reflexes ____________________ Tremor ____________________

Genital and Anal Examination

Details of Female Genital Findings

Site Examined	Findings *(Bleeding/ tear/ discharge/ edema/ tenderness)*
Thighs	
Mons pubis, perineal tear	
Pubic hair (matted, shaved, cut)	
Labia majora	
Labia minora	
Clitoris	
Fourchette	
Fossa navicularis	
Vestibule	
Urethra	
Hymen (edges, position of tear)	
Posterior commissure	

Internal findings (if applicable)

Vaginal wall ____________________

Cervix ____________________

Details of Anal Findings

Natal fold	
Perianal/ anal margin	
Internal findings	

Specific Examinations *(wherever facilities exists, and if indicated)*

a. Toluidine blue dye test ____________________

b. Per speculum findings, if performed* ____________________

c. Per vaginum findings, if performed* ____________________

d. Wet mount slide test ____________________

e. UV light examination of clothes and skin ____________________

f. Colposcopic/ Proctoscopic examination ____________________

* Per vaginum/ per speculum examination should not be done unless required for detection of injuries or for medical treatment.

Details of Male Genital Findings

Site	Findings *(Bleeding/ tear/ discharge/ edema/ tenderness)*
Thighs	
Pubic area	
Pubic hair	
Scrotum	
Testes	
Penis	
Foreskin	

Sample Collected/ Investigations for Hospital/ Clinical Laboratory

(Tick '✓')

☐ Blood for HIV, VDRL, HbsAg

☐ Urine test for pregnancy

☐ Ultrasound for pregnancy/ internal injury

☐ X-ray/ CT for injury

Samples Collected for Forensic Science Laboratory

(Samples to be packed, sealed and labeled separately. Swab sticks should be moistened with distilled water)

1. Debris collection paper
2. Clothing evidence where available (to be packed in separate paper bags after air drying)

Body evidence samples, as appropriate (duly labeled and packed separately)

Samples	Collected/ Not Collected	Reason(s) for not collecting
Swabs from stains on the body		
Scalp hair (10–15 strands)		
Head hair combing		
Nail scrapings/ clippings (both hands)		
Oral swab		
Blood for grouping (plain vial)		
Blood for drug/ alcohol levels (sodium fluoride vial)		
Blood for DNA analysis (EDTA vial/ FTA card)		
Urine (drug testing)		
Any other (tampon/ sanitary napkin/ condom/ object)		

Genital and Anal Evidence

Samples	Collected/ Not Collected	Reason(s) for not collecting
Matted pubic hair		
Pubic hair combing and cutting (mention, if shaved)		
Two vulval swabs (for semen and DNA testing)		
Two vaginal swabs (for semen and DNA testing)		
Two anal swabs (for semen and DNA testing)		
Vaginal smear (air-dried) for semen examination		
Vaginal washing		
Urethral swab		
Swab from clitoris/ glans of penis		

*Samples to be preserved in refrigerator till handed over to police along with duly attested sample seal

Treatment prescribed ____________________

Time of completion of examination ____________________

Provisional Medical Opinion

I have examined (name of survivor) ____________________ aged about __________ years reporting with alleged history of (type of sexual violence and circumstances) ____________________

____________________ after __________ (days/ hours) of the incident. My findings are as follows:

- Important clinical findings ____________________
- Additional observations (if any) ____________________
- Samples collected (for FSL), awaiting reports ____________________
- Samples collected (for hospital laboratory) ____________________

On the basis of above mentioned observations, I am of the opinion that *(Refer to Table 5.1)* ____________________

____

____

Place __________

Date __________

____
Signature of the Doctor
Name, Designation and Seal

Copy of the entire medical report must be given to the survivor free of cost immediately

This report contains .... number of sheets and .... number of envelopes and .... number of samples.

Received MLR No. __________ along with body diagram and __________ number of envelopes, __________ number of samples and sample seal.

Name ____________________ P.C. No. __________ P.S. __________

____
Signature and date

Date __________ **MLR No.** __________ **CR No.** __________

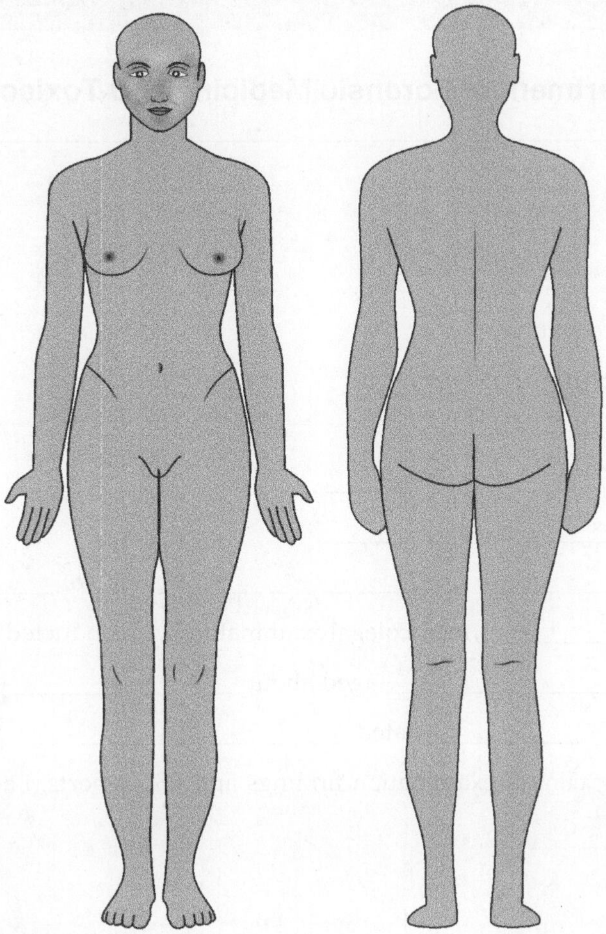

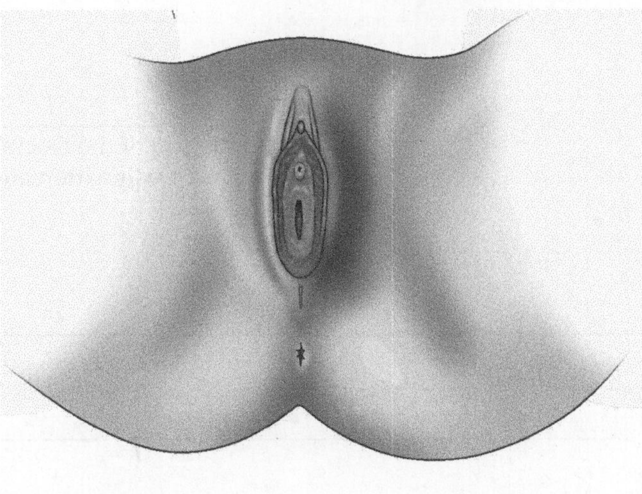

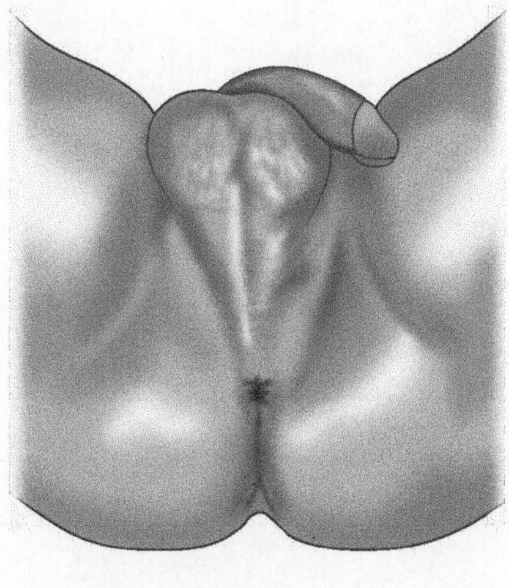

Signature of the Doctor
Name, Designation and Seal

EX. 5.2: FINAL OPINION REGARDING VICTIM OF SEXUAL VIOLENCE (Rape)

Department of Forensic Medicine and Toxicology

____

To Date ___________

The Investigating Officer,

____________________ Police Station

____________________ (District/ City/ Town)

Ref:

a. FSL report no. ____________________ dated ________

b. Toxicology report no. __________ dated ________

As per requisition from the ______________________________________ of ____________________________

police station dated ____________________, medicolegal examination was conducted on ______________________

D/ W of ________________________________ aged about _______________ years, gender ______________,

and the MLR number ____________________ dated ________________________ was issued by the undersigned.

Taking into account the history, clinical examination findings and FSL reports, I am of the opinion that: *(Refer to Table 5.1)*

____

Signature of the Doctor
Name, Designation and Seal

Place _________

Date _________

Received final opinion regarding MLR No. _____________ dated __________.

Name ______________________________ P.C. No. __________________________ P.S. _________________

____

Signature and date

EX. 5.3: EXAMINATION OF ACCUSED OF SEXUAL VIOLENCE (Rape/ Sodomy)

Mukesh Singh, a 37-year-old male was brought by the police with alleged history of raping his neighbor. He is well built, 179 cm tall and weighed 78 kg. The incident took place 6.00 to 7.00 PM and the police arrested him from his friend's place at 12 midnight and brought him for examination. Prepare a medicolegal report for the same.

Department of Forensic Medicine and Toxicology

____

MLR No. ________________ C.R. No. ________

Patient Details

Name ________________________________ Son of ________________________

Address ____

Age (as reported) ______ years Date of birth (if known) ________________

Gender ________________ Marital status: Unmarried/ Married/ Divorced

Examination Details

Date and Time of examination________________

Requisition from ________________________ Vide letter no. ____________ Dated ________

Brought by (Name and signature) ________________________ P.C. No.__________ P.S.__________

Informed Consent

(Consent is asked for, but if refused, reasonable force may be used if examination is done under Sec. 53 A CrPC)

I, ________________________________Son of ________________________________

hereby give my consent for examination and sample collection for medicolegal examination, knowing that the result of the examination may go in my favor or against.

I understand that the examination will include:
- A full medical history and complete examination (including examination of genital organs);
- Collection of forensic specimens;
- Taking of photographs/ digital images for recording and evidential purposes;
- I understand and agree that a copy of the medical notes may be given to professionals involved in the case (e.g. police or lawyers) and may be used in the court;
- I agree to the use of my anonymized photographs/ digital images/ medical notes for teaching, audit and research.

The above have been explained to me in ________________________ language which I can understand.

Date____________

Name and signature (thumb impression)
of the examinee

Marks of Identification

1. ______________________________

2. ______________________________

Brief history of assault as stated by the accused (use separate sheet, if necessary) ______________________________

____

____

____

Did the accused know the victim before? ☐ No ☐ Yes If yes, relationship ______________________________

Medical History and Allergies

General health ______________________________

Pre-existing skin problems, e.g. eczema, lichen sclerosus ______________________________

Prescribed medication ______________________________

Vaccination status: Hepatitis B (Vaccinated/ Not vaccinated)

Allergies ______________________________

DETAILS OF THE ASSAULT FROM EXAMINEE

Specific Information Relating to the Alleged Offence

Date and time of assault ____________________ Time interval to examination ____________________

Type of surface where assault occurred ______________________________

Query	*Tick '√'*	Details
Kissing/ licking/ biting/ sucking/ spitting (*sites*)	☐ Not Known ☐ No ☐ Yes	
Penile-oral penetration	☐ Not Known ☐ No ☐ Yes	
Penile-anal penetration	☐ Not Known ☐ No ☐ Yes	
Penile-vaginal penetration	☐ Not Known ☐ No ☐ Yes	
Digital penetration	☐ Not Known ☐ No ☐ Yes	
Mouth to genitalia/ anus	☐ Not Known ☐ No ☐ Yes	
Object to vulva/ vagina/ anus	☐ Not Known ☐ No ☐ Yes	
Other sexual/ physical act(s)	☐ Not Known ☐ No ☐ Yes	
Ejaculation onto skin/ hair	☐ Not Known ☐ No ☐ Yes	
Condom used throughout	☐ Not Known ☐ No ☐ Yes	
Lubricant/ spermicide used	☐ Not Known ☐ No ☐ Yes	
Injuries inflicted	☐ Not Known ☐ No ☐ Yes	
Damage to clothing	☐ Not Known ☐ No ☐ Yes	

Threat Used During Assault

a. Physical violence *(Tick '√')*

☐ Hit with hand, fist, blunt object, sharp object	☐ Bitten	☐ Pulled hair
☐ Burned	☐ Kicked	☐ Pinched
☐ Violently shaken	☐ Head banged	☐ Dragged

b. Emotional abuse (insulting, cursing, belittling, terrorizing) ____________________

c. Use of restraints, if any ____________________

d. Used weapon(s) or objects, if any ____________________

e. Verbal threats, if any: ____________________

f. Luring (sweets, chocolates, money or job), if any: ____________________

g. Any other ____________________

If survivor has injured the accused (details) ____________________

Post Assault

Genital/ relevant skin: Wiped/ washed Specify site and disposal of cloth/ tissue	☐ Not Known ☐ No ☐ Yes ____________________
Passed urine	☐ Not Known ☐ No ☐ Yes (note time)
Oral intercourse: Drank/ eaten food	☐ Not Known ☐ No ☐ Yes
Anal intercourse: Defecated since offence	☐ Not Known ☐ No ☐ Yes
Changed/ washed clothes If changed, are the clothes available?	☐ Not Known ☐ No ☐ Yes ☐ No ☐ Yes
Cleaned/ washed undergarments	☐ Not Known ☐ No ☐ Yes
Taken bath/ shower	☐ Not Known ☐ No ☐ Yes

Drug and Alcohol use in Relation to Assault

Was alcohol consumed? ☐ Not Known ☐ No ☐ Yes

If yes, please specify ☐ Post Offence ☐ Prior ☐ During

Start time of drinking ____________________ End time of drinking ____________________

Quantity and type of beverage consumed ____________________

Any illicit drugs been used within 4 days of the examination? ☐ Not Known ☐ No ☐ Yes

If yes, specify ☐ Post Offence ☐ Prior ☐ During

Give details ____________________

General Examination

Clothes

- Foreign matter/ Stains: Blood/ seminal/ fecal/ mud/ lipstick/ hair/ grass/ any other ______________________
- Buttons/ zipper: Intact/ undone/ broken/ torn

Built: Well/ Average/ Poor Height ______ cm Weight ______ kg

Pulse _______/ min BP __________ mm Hg Respiratory rate _____/ min

General appearance ____

Signs of intoxication ____

Demeanor/ behavior ☐ Sober ☐ Excited ☐ Terrified ☐ Calm ☐ Depressed

Speech (e.g. content, form) ____

Secondary sexual characters ____

Injuries (type, site, size, shape, color, swelling and signs of healing)/ Scar/ Stains/ Foreign body

Site Examined		Injuries	Type of injury	Features/ Remarks
Face		☐ No ☐ Yes		
Eyes		☐ No ☐ Yes		
Lips		☐ No ☐ Yes		
Teeth		☐ No ☐ Yes		
Neck		☐ No ☐ Yes		
Back		☐ No ☐ Yes		
Arms	Right Left	☐ No ☐ Yes ☐ No ☐ Yes		
Hands/ wrists	Right Left	☐ No ☐ Yes ☐ No ☐ Yes		
Fingers/ nails	Right Left	☐ No ☐ Yes ☐ No ☐ Yes		
Front of chest		☐ No ☐ Yes		
Abdomen		☐ No ☐ Yes		
Additional details				

(Tick '✓')

Systemic Examination ____

____

Genital Examination

General development ____________________

Site Examined	Findings *(stains/ foreign body/ bleeding/ tear/ edema/ tenderness)*
Thighs	
Pubic area	
Pubic hair (matted/ shaved/ cut)	
Scrotum	
Testes	
Prepuce	Retractable/ Nonretractable/ Circumcised
Smegma (retract prepuce and observe)	Present/ Absent
Frenulum	Torn/ Intact
Penis (any deformity, abrasion, smell)	
Signs of sexually transmitted disease (discharge)	

Specific Examination *(if done)*

Lugol's iodine test ____________________

Sample Collected/ Investigations for Hospital Laboratory

1. Blood for HIV, VDRL, HbsAg, WR and Kahn test
2. X-ray/ CT for injury

Samples Collected for Forensic Science Laboratory

(Samples to be packed, sealed and labeled separately. Swab sticks should be moistened with distilled water)

1. Debris collection paper
2. Clothing evidence, where available (to be packed in separate paper bags after air drying)

Body evidence samples, as appropriate (duly labeled and packed separately)

Samples	Collected/ Not Collected	Reason(s) for not collecting
Swabs from stains on the body/ teeth bite		
Scalp hair (10–15 strands)		
Nail scrapings/ clippings (both hands)		
Blood for grouping (plain vial)		
Blood for drug/ alcohol levels (sodium fluoride vial)		
Blood for DNA analysis (EDTA vial/ FTA card)		
Urine (drug testing)		
Any other (e.g. swab from discharge, lubricant)		

Genital Evidence

Samples	Collected/ Not Collected	Reason(s) for not collecting
Matted pubic hair		
Pubic hair combing and cutting (mention, if shaved)		
Prostatic swab for gonorrheal secretions		
Swab from prepuce, coronal sulcus (vaginal cells/ fecal matter)		

*Samples to be preserved in refrigerator till handed over to police along with duly attested sample seal

Time of completion of examination ____________________

Provisional Medical Opinion

Taking into consideration the history of the case and clinical examination, I am of the opinion that:

- ☐ The possibility of recent performance of sexual intercourse cannot be ruled out, i.e. there is evidence of recent penetration of vagina/ anus. However, final opinion will be given after receiving the FSL report.
- ☐ The examinee is incapable of performing sexual intercourse in the ordinary way or accomplish penetration (gross penile deformity).

(Tick '✓')

Place ____________ Signature of the Doctor

Date ____________ Name, Designation and Seal

Received MLR No. ________ along with body diagram and ________ number of envelopes, ________ number of samples and sample seal.

Name ____________________ P.C. No. ____________ P.S. ____________

Signature and date

Date ___________ **MLR No.** ___________ **CR No.** ___________

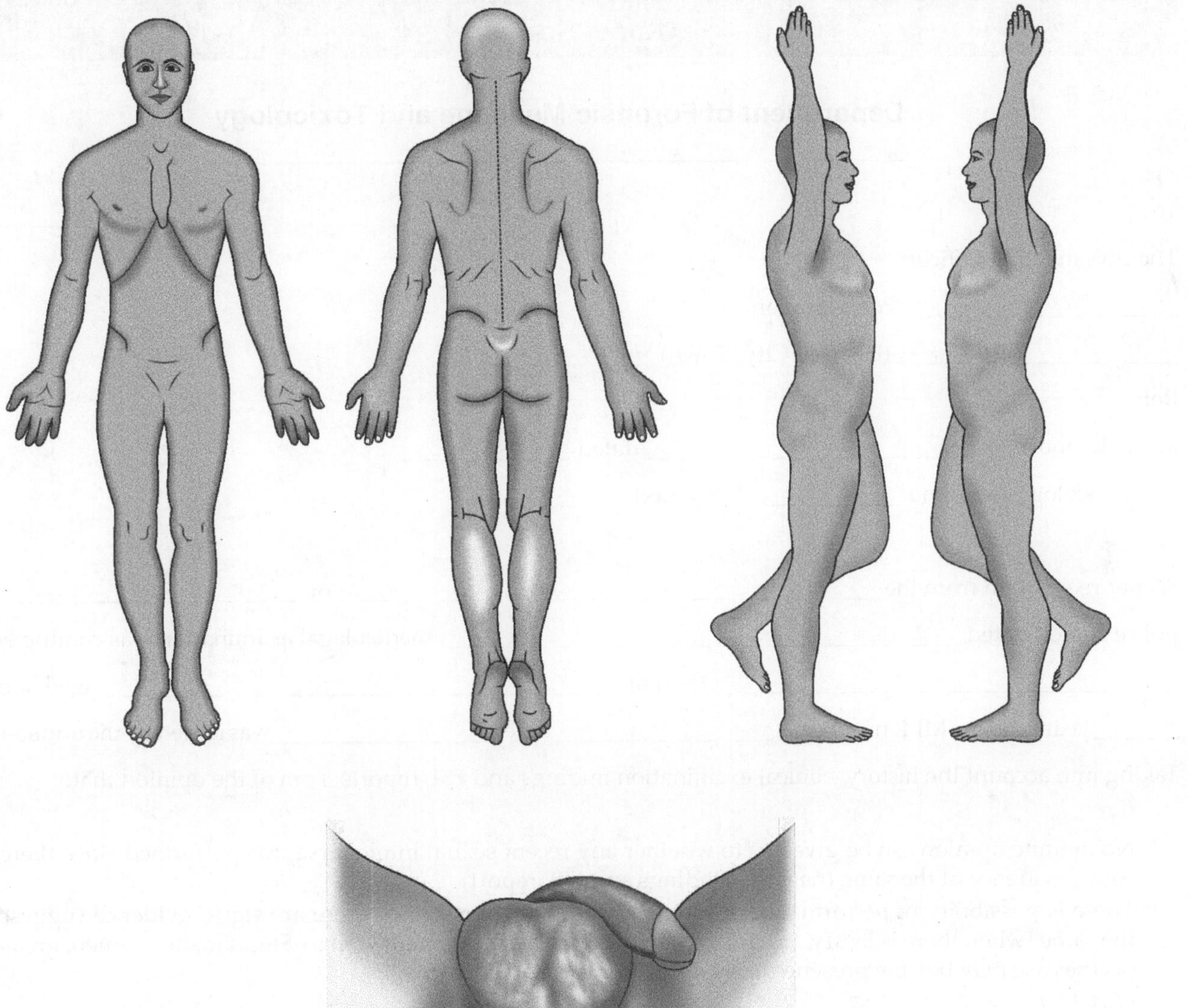

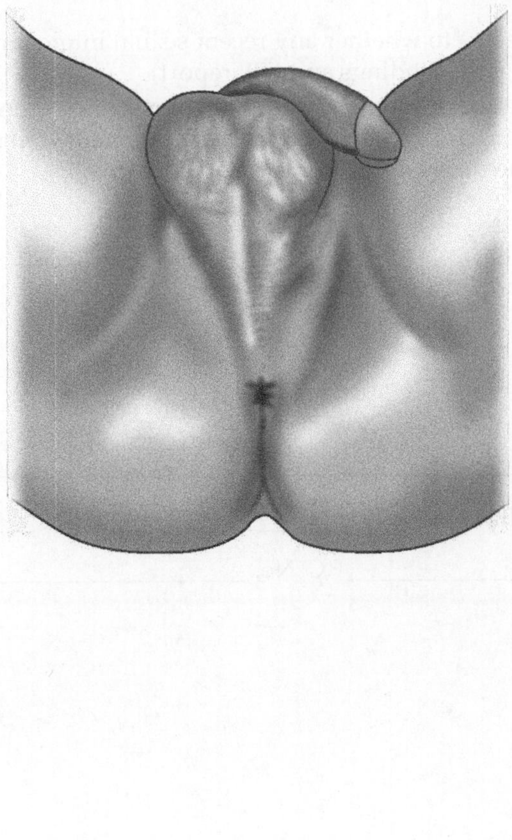

Signature of the Doctor
Name, Designation and Seal

EX. 5.4: FINAL OPINION REGARDING ACCUSED OF SEXUAL VIOLENCE (Rape/ Sodomy)

Department of Forensic Medicine and Toxicology

____

To Date ____________

The Investigating Officer,

______________________Police Station

______________________ (District/ City/ Town)

Ref:

a. FSL report no. __________________________ dated _____________

b. Toxicology report no. _______________ dated __________

As per requisition from the ____ of ____________________________ police station dated ____, medicolegal examination was conducted on ______________________________________ Son of ____ aged about _______ years and the MLR number __________________ dated ________________ was issued by the undersigned.

Taking into account the history, clinical examination findings and FSL reports, I am of the opinion that:

- ☐ No definite opinion can be given as to whether any recent sexual intercourse was performed since there is no signs/ evidence of the same (negative findings and FSL report)
- ☐ There is possibility of performance of recent sexual intercourse since there are signs/ evidence suggestive of the same [when there is injury, FSL report show vaginal epithelium or stains of fecal matter, semen, grease, etc. (as the case may be); the presence of injury on penis is corroborative]

(Tick '✓')

____

Signature of the Doctor

Place ________________ Name, Designation and Seal

Date _________________

Received final opinion regarding MLR No. ______________________ dated _______________________ .

Name ____________________________________ P.C. No. _______________________ P.S. ______________________

____

Signature and date

EX. 5.5: EXAMINATION OF VICTIM OF UNNATURAL SEXUAL VIOLENCE

Manish Ranawat, a 13-year-old boy was allegedly sodomised by his acquaintance after luring him to a lonely spot while they were playing cricket. There he forcefully made him sleep on ground and had unnatural sex and later forced him to clean up. He also threatened the victim with death threats to keep quiet about the act. His parents complained to the police who brought the victim for examination. Prepare a report for the same.

Department of Forensic Medicine and Toxicology

____

MLR No. ______________ C.R. No. ______________

Patient Details

Name ____ S/ D/ W of ____________________

Address ____

Age (as reported) ______ years Date of birth (if known) ______________

Gender________________ Marital status: Unmarried/ Married/ Divorced

Examination Details

Date and Time of examination____________________

Requisition from ______________________________ Vide letter no. ______________ Dated __________

Brought by (Name and signature) ________________________ P.C. No.____________ P.S.____________

Informed Consent

I, ____________________________________ S/ D/ W of ______________________________________

hereby give my consent for examination and sample collection for medicolegal examination, knowing that the result of the examination may go in my favor or against.

I understand that the examination will include:

- A full medical history and complete examination (including examination of genital organs);
- Collection of forensic specimens;
- Taking of photographs/ digital images for recording and evidential purposes;
- I understand and agree that a copy of the medical notes may be given to professionals involved in the case (e.g. police or lawyers) and may be used in the court;
- I agree to the use of my anonymized photographs/ digital images/ medical notes for teaching, audit and research.

The above have been explained to me in ________________________________ language which I can understand.

Date____________

Name and signature (thumb impression)
of the examinee

Marks of Identification

1. ____________________

2. ____________________

History

As given by police ____________________

Brief history of assault as stated by the accused (use separate sheet, if necessary) ____________________

____

____

____

Did the accused know the victim before? ☐ No ☐ Yes If yes, relationship ____________________

Medical History and Allergies

General health ____________________

Pre-existing skin problems, e.g. eczema, lichen sclerosus ____________________

Prescribed medication ____________________

Vaccination status: Hepatitis B (Vaccinated/ Not vaccinated)

Allergies ____________________

DETAILS OF THE ASSAULT FROM EXAMINEE

Specific Information Relating to the Alleged Offence

Date and time of assault ____________________ Time interval to examination ____________________

Whether sleeping or unconscious during the act? ____________________

Whether cried for help or struggled or resisted? ____________________

Query	*Tick '√'*	Details
Kissing/ licking/ biting/ sucking/ spitting *(sites)*	☐ Not Known ☐ No ☐ Yes	
Penile-oral penetration	☐ Not Known ☐ No ☐ Yes	
Penile-anal penetration	☐ Not Known ☐ No ☐ Yes	
Penile-vaginal penetration	☐ Not Known ☐ No ☐ Yes	
Digital penetration	☐ Not Known ☐ No ☐ Yes	
Mouth to genitalia/ anus	☐ Not Known ☐ No ☐ Yes	
Object to vulva/ vagina/ anus	☐ Not Known ☐ No ☐ Yes	
Other sexual/ physical act(s)	☐ Not Known ☐ No ☐ Yes	
Ejaculation onto skin/ hair	☐ Not Known ☐ No ☐ Yes	

Condom used throughout	☐ Not Known ☐ No ☐ Yes	
Lubricant/ spermicide used	☐ Not Known ☐ No ☐ Yes	
Injuries inflicted	☐ Not Known ☐ No ☐ Yes	
Damage to clothing	☐ Not Known ☐ No ☐ Yes	

Threat Used During Assault

a. Physical violence *(Tick '√')*

☐ Hit with hand, fist, blunt object, sharp object	☐ Bitten	☐ Pulled hair
☐ Burned	☐ Kicked	☐ Pinched
☐ Violently shaken	☐ Head banged	☐ Dragged

b. Emotional abuse (insulting, cursing, belittling, terrorizing) ____________________

c. Use of restraints, if any ____________________

d. Used weapon(s) or objects, if any ____________________

e. Verbal threats, if any: ____________________

f. Luring (sweets, chocolates, money or job), if any: ____________________

g. Any other ____________________

If survivor has injured the accused (details) ____________________

Post Assault

Genital/ relevant skin: Wiped/ washed Specify site and disposal of cloth/ tissue	☐ Not Known ☐ No ☐ Yes ____________________
Passed urine	☐ Not Known ☐ No ☐ Yes (note time)
Oral intercourse: Drank/ eaten food	☐ Not Known ☐ No ☐ Yes
Anal intercourse: Defecated since offence	☐ Not Known ☐ No ☐ Yes
Changed/ washed clothes If changed, are the clothes available?	☐ Not Known ☐ No ☐ Yes ☐ No ☐ Yes
Cleaned/ washed undergarments	☐ Not Known ☐ No ☐ Yes
Taken bath/ shower	☐ Not Known ☐ No ☐ Yes

Drug and Alcohol use in Relation to Assault

Was alcohol consumed? ☐ Not Known ☐ No ☐ Yes

If yes, please specify ☐ Post Offence ☐ Prior ☐ During

Start time of drinking ____________________ End time of drinking ____________________

Quantity and type of beverage consumed ____________________

Any illicit drugs been used within 4 days of the examination? ☐ Not Known ☐ No ☐ Yes

If yes, specify ☐ Post Offence ☐ Prior ☐ During

Give details ____________________

General Examination

Clothes

- Foreign matter/ Stains: Blood/ seminal/ fecal/ mud/ hair/ grass/ any other ____________
- Buttons/ zipper: Intact/ undone/ broken/ torn

Built: Well/ Average/ Poor Height _______ cm Weight _______ kg

Pulse ________/ min BP ___________ mm Hg Respiratory rate ______/ min

General appearance ____________________

Signs of intoxication ____________________

Demeanor/ behavior ☐ Sober ☐ Excited ☐ Terrified ☐ Calm ☐ Depressed

Speech (e.g. content, form) ____________________

Secondary sexual characters ____________________

Injuries (type, site, size, shape, color, swelling and signs of healing)/ Scar/ Stains/ Foreign body

Site Examined		Injuries		Type of injury	Features/ Remarks
Face		☐ No	☐ Yes		
Eyes		☐ No	☐ Yes		
Lips		☐ No	☐ Yes		
Teeth		☐ No	☐ Yes		
Neck		☐ No	☐ Yes		
Back		☐ No	☐ Yes		
Arms	Right Left	☐ No ☐ No	☐ Yes ☐ Yes		
Hands/ wrists	Right Left	☐ No ☐ No	☐ Yes ☐ Yes		
Fingers/ nails	Right Left	☐ No ☐ No	☐ Yes ☐ Yes		
Front of chest		☐ No	☐ Yes		
Abdomen		☐ No	☐ Yes		
Additional details					

(Tick '✓')

Systemic Examination ____________________

____

Genital Examination

General development ____________________

Site Examined	Findings *(stains/ foreign body/ bleeding/ tear/ edema/ tenderness)*
Thighs	
Pubic area	
Pubic hair (matted/ shaved/ cut)	
Signs of sexually transmitted disease	
Natal fold	
Perianal/ anal margin	
Anus	Anal mucosa ☐ Smooth ☐ Thickened Tears ☐ Present ☐ Absent If present: Recent/ Old Depression of anus ☐ Present ☐ Not present Hemorrhoids ☐ Present ☐ Not present Stains of blood/ semen/ lubricants ☐ Present ☐ Absent
Anal sphincter	Tone ☐ Retained ☐ Lost Rugal pattern ☐ Retained ☐ Lost Lateral traction test ☐ Orifice closes ☐ Relaxes reflexly Per rectal Admits one/ more finger, with/ without pain
Rectum	

Speculum examination ____________________

Sample Collected/ Investigations for Hospital Laboratory

1. Blood for HIV, VDRL, HbsAg
2. X-ray/ CT for injury

Samples Collected for Forensic Science Laboratory

(Samples to be packed, sealed and labeled separately. Swab sticks should be moistened with distilled water)

1. Debris collection paper
2. Clothing evidence, where available (to be packed in separate paper bags after air drying)

Body evidence samples, as appropriate (duly labeled and packed separately)

Samples	Collected/ Not Collected	Reason(s) for not collecting
Swabs from stains on the body/ teeth bite		
Scalp hair (10–15 strands)		
Buccal swabs		
Nail scrapings/ clippings (both hands)		
Blood for grouping (plain vial)		
Blood for drug/ alcohol levels (sodium fluoride vial)		
Blood for DNA analysis (EDTA vial/ FTA card)		
Urine (drug testing)		
Any other (e.g. swab from discharge, lubricant)		

Genital Evidence

Samples	Collected/ Not Collected	Reason(s) for not collecting
Matted pubic hair		
Pubic hair combing and cutting (mention, if shaved)		
Anal swabs		
Loose hair from anal region and buttocks		

*Samples to be preserved in refrigerator till handed over to police along with duly attested sample seal

Time of completion of examination ____________________

Provisional Medical Opinion

On the basis of above mentioned observations, I am of the opinion that the findings of examination is consistent with/ not inconsistent with the history of alleged sexual intercourse, i.e. there is evidence of/ no evidence of recent penetration of anus/ buccal coitus. However, final opinion will be given after receiving of FSL report.

Place ____________ Signature of the Doctor

Date ____________ Name, Designation and Seal

Received MLR no. ____________ along with body diagram and ____________ number of envelopes, ____________ number of samples and sample seal.

Name ____________ P.C. No. ____________ P.S. ____________

Signature and date

Date ___________ **MLR No.** ___________ **CR No.** ___________

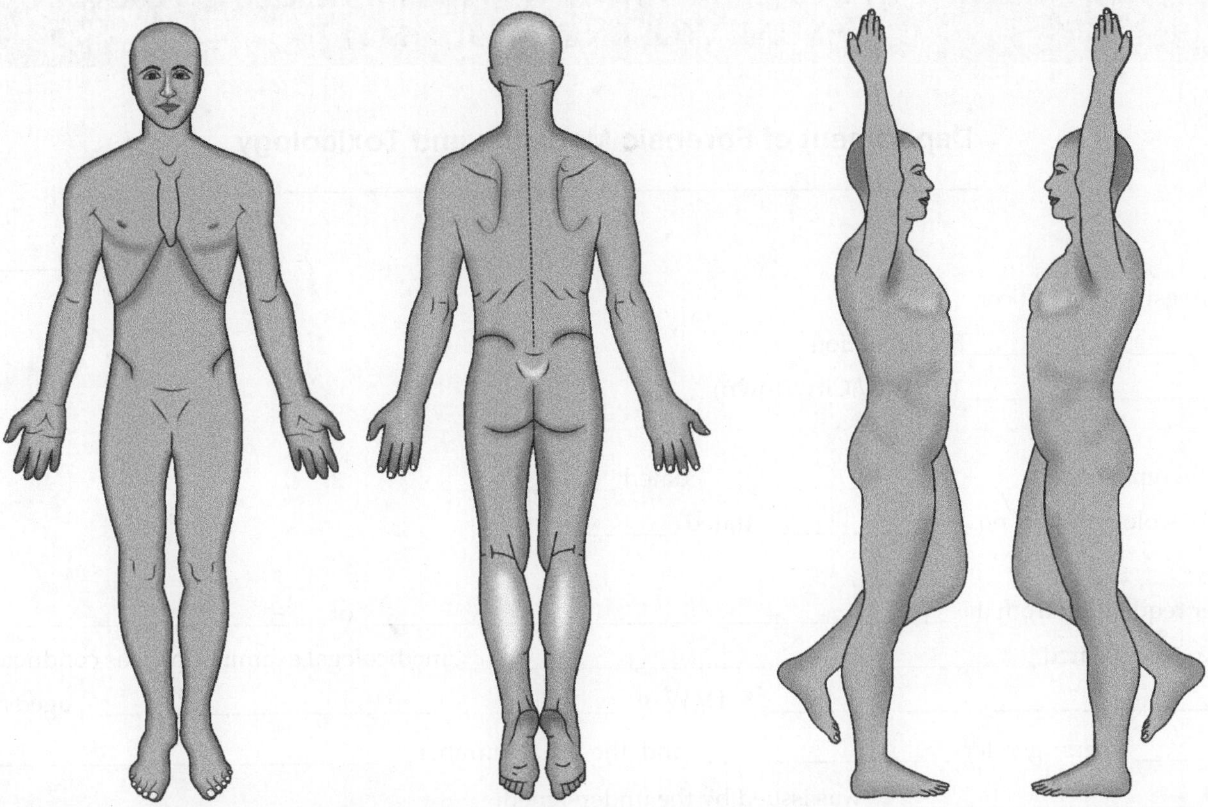

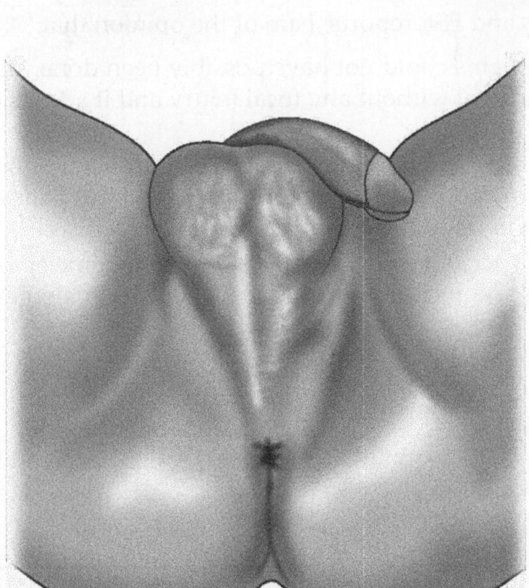

____
Signature of the Doctor
Name, Designation and Seal

EX. 5.6: FINAL OPINION REGARDING VICTIM OF UNNATURAL SEXUAL VIOLENCE (SODOMY)

Department of Forensic Medicine and Toxicology

____

To Date ____________

The Investigating Officer,

____________________Police Station

____________________ (District/ City/ Town)

Ref:

a. FSL report no. ______________________ dated ____________

b. Toxicology report no. ______________ dated _________

As per requisition from the ______________________________ of ________________ police station dated ______________________________, medicolegal examination was conducted on ______________________________ S/ D/ W of ______________________________ aged about ________ years, gender ______________, and the MLR number ____________________ dated ____________________ was issued by the undersigned.

Taking into account the history, clinical examination findings and FSL reports, I am of the opinion that:

- ☐ Full act of anal sexual intercourse by normal sized adult penis could not have possibly been done, since there are no signs of recent or past penetration (if the anus is normal without any focal injury and it admits only one finger without difficulty with or without lubricant)
- ☐ A recent full act of anal sexual intercourse with a full sized erect adult penis has in all probability been done since there are signs of recent anal penetration (if anus admits one or two fingers with or without pain, evidence of fresh tear or bruise around the anal margin along with evidence of seminal emission.)
- ☐ The subject is a habituated to anal intercourse and is well accustomed to such acts for some time since past (if the anal sphincter is loose and lax, anal canal is patulous and rectum is visible through well dilated anal canal or anus showing funnel shaped depression).

(Tick '✓')

____

Signature of the Doctor
Name, Designation and Seal

Place ______________

Date ______________

Received final opinion regarding MLR No. ____________________ dated ______________ .

Name________________________ P.C.No.________________________ P.S.________________

____

Signature and date

Ex. 5.7: EXAMINATION OF A CASE OF IMPOTENCY

Rehman Malik, a 45-year-old unemployed man, accused of rape and abduction, was brought for examination of potency. He is charged with raping of a 16-year-old girl and has been in custody for the last 1 month. He pleaded not guilty before the court citing impotence. The court ordered the accused to undergo potency test. Prepare a report regarding the same.

Department of Forensic Medicine and Toxicology

____

MLR No. ______________ C.R. No. ____________

Patient Details

Name ______________________ S/ D/ W of ______________________

Address ______________________________ Gender ____________

Age (as reported) ________ years Date of birth (if known) ____________

Marital status: Unmarried/ Married/ Divorced If married, number of children ________

Occupation ____________________ Educational status ____________________

Examination Details

Date and Time of examination ______________________________

Requisition from ____________________ Vide letter no. __________ Dated ________

Brought by (Name and signature) ____________________ P.C. No.__________ P.S.__________

Accompanied by (name and relation) ______________________________

Informed Consent

I, ______________________ S/ D/ W of ______________________ hereby agree for a complete physical examination (including examination of genital organs), recording of findings, collection of specimens as necessary for laboratory analysis, photographic documentation and any other investigations as recommended by the examining doctor and release of a report to the police officials/ court of law concerned. This procedure has been fully explained to me. Further, I have been explained that the result may go against me. This information may be used for teaching and research purposes, provided no identifying data is released.

The above has been explained to me in ____________language and I have fully understood the same and I am signing this consent by my own free will.

______________ ______________

Signature and name of the witness Signature/ Thumb impression of the examinee

Address ______________

Marks of Identification

1. ______________________________

2. ______________________________

Brief history of the case ______________________________

____

____

History and Allergies

General health ______________________________

Developmental abnormalities ______________________________

Past illness ______________________________

Local/ General disease ______________________________

Occupational history ______________________________

Previous trauma (especially spine) ______________________________

Prescribed medication ______________________________

Drug/ Addiction ______________________________

Smoking/ Alcohol ______________________________

Allergies ______________________________

Sexual history ______________________________

Specific enquiry (males)

Morning erection of penis ______________________________

Night emissions ______________________________

Attitude towards opposite sex ______________________________

Masturbation (frequency) ______________________________

Psychosocial history ______________________________

____

General Examination

Built: Well/ Average/ Poor   Height ________ cm   Weight ________ kg

Pulse ________/ min   BP ________ mm Hg   Respiratory rate ________/ min

General appearance ______________________________

Demeanor/ behavior ☐ Sober ☐ Eccentric ☐ Erratic ☐ Calm ☐ Depressed

Hair: Pubic/ axillary/ facial/ chest/ scalp (male/ female type hair line)

Secondary sexual characters ______________________________

Systemic Examination

CVS Examination (for signs of atherosclerosis) ______________________________

Respiratory System Examination ______________________________

GIT Examination ______________________________

CNS Examination (pain, touch vibration and other sensations) ______________________________

Cranial Nerve Examination ______________________________

Reflexes ______________________________

Spine ______________________________

Peripheral Vascular System ______________________________

Local Examination

In case of male

A. Penis	
Present/ Absent	
Length and circumference Flaccid Erect	
Development	
Disease	
Deformity	
Discharge	
Injury	
Bulbocavernosus reflex	Positive/ Negative
Prepuce	Retractable/ Nonretractable/ Circumcised
Urethral orifice	Normal/ Glandular/ Coronal/ Penile shaft/ Scrotal/ Perineal
Smegma	Present/ Absent
Hygiene	
B. Scrotum	Pendulous/ Nonpendulous
C. Testes	
Size Right Left	Infantile/ Adult/ Enlarged/ Atrophied/ Absent Infantile/ Adult/ Enlarged/ Atrophied/ Absent
Epididymis/ Spermatic cord	
Cremasteric reflex	

In Case of Female

A. Vulva	
Clitoris (size)	
Infections	
Tumors	
B. Vagina	
Sensation	Hyperesthesia/ Normal
Congenital defects	
Infections	
Tumors	
C. Cervix	
Congenital anomalies	
Tumors/ Carcinoma	
D. Uterus and appendages	
Congenital anomalies	
Tenderness	
Disease	
Adnexal masses	
Infections	

Sample Collected/ Investigative

1. Blood, urine, semen (in males), and Pap smear from cervix (in females).
2. X-ray of chest, skull, spine

Potency Tests *(in males)*

1. Injection of PGE1 ____________________
2. Duplex Ultrasonography ____________________
3. Ultrasonography of testes ____________________
4. Noctural penile tumescence ____________________
5. Penile biothesiometry ____________________

Opinion

From the above examination and tests, I am of the opinion that:

☐ There is nothing to suggest that the person is incapable of performing sexual intercourse.

☐ The person is incapable of performing sexual intercourse due to ______________________. (for example, there is evidence of disease of central nervous system which may cause impairment of sexual activity)

(Tick '✓')

Place __________ ______________________
Signature of the Doctor

Date __________ Name, Designation and Seal

Received MLR No. ____________ along with ____________ number of envelopes and ____________ number of samples and sample seal.

Name ______________________ P.C. No. ____________ P.S. ____________

____
Signature and date

NOTES

NOTES

NOTES

UNIT VI

Death Certification

The **name of deceased** is written in full. Do not use initials. If deceased is an infant, not yet named at time of death, write, 'Son of (S/o) or Daughter of (D/o)', followed by names of mother and father.

Cause of Death

The certificate of cause of death is divided into two parts, I and II.

Part I is again divided into three parts, lines (a) (b) (c). If a single morbid condition completely explains the death, then this will be written on line (a) of Part I, and nothing more need to be written in the rest of Part I or in Part II. Often, however, a number of morbid conditions may have been present at death. If so, enter the antecedent causes in Part I, line (b)—the disease or injury that initiated the chain of morbid events that led directly and inevitably to death. Sometimes, there may be three stages in the course of events leading to death. If so, line (c) should be completed. The underlying cause to be tabulated is always written last in Part I.

- First enter in Part I (a) the immediate cause of death (the final disease, injury, or complication directly causing death). *The cause-of-death information should be the best medical opinion.* Abbreviation should not be used. Two or more conditions should not be written on a single line. A condition can be listed as 'probable' even if it has not been definitively diagnosed.
- The mode of dying, e.g. cardiac arrest, respiratory arrest or ventricular fibrillation should not be used without showing the etiology. These terms should not appear on the certificate at all since they are modes of dying and not causes of death. If a mechanism of death seems most appropriate for (a), then list its cause(s) on the line(s) below it (e.g. cardiac arrest **due to** coronary artery atherosclerosis or cardiac arrest **due to** blunt impact to chest).
- If an organ system failure such as congestive heart failure, hepatic failure, renal failure or respiratory failure is listed as a cause of death, always report its etiology on the line(s) beneath it (e.g. renal failure **due to** Type I diabetes mellitus).

Part II *(Other significant conditions):* Enter all diseases or conditions contributing to death that were not reported in the chain of events in Part I and that did not result in the **underlying cause of death.**

Onset: For each cause, indicate the best estimate of the interval between the presumed onset and the date of death. The terms 'unknown' or 'approximately' (e.g. 'from birth', 'several years') may be used. General terms, such as minutes, hours or days are acceptable, if necessary.

Maternal deaths: This information is needed for all women of child-bearing age, even though the pregnancy may have had nothing to do with the death.

Old age or senility: Old age (or senility) should be not given as a cause of death if a more specific cause is known. If old age was contributory factor, it should be entered in Part II.

Manner of Death

Always mention the manner of death since it is important:

a. In determining accurate causes of death
b. In processing insurance claims
c. In statistical studies of injuries and death.

Indicate 'could not be determined' **ONLY** when it is impossible to determine the manner of death.

The following conditions and types of death might seem to be specific or natural but when the medical history is examined further may be found to be complications of an injury or poisoning (possibly occurring long ago). Such cases should be reported to the police.

Epidural/ subarachnoid/ subdural hematoma	Thermal burns/ chemical burns	Open reduction of fracture
Exsanguination	Choking	Drug or alcohol overdose
Fall	Fracture/ Hip fracture	Asphyxia
Pulmonary emboli	Hyper-/ hypothermia	Surgery
Seizure disorder	Bolus	Sepsis

EX. 6.1: MEDICAL CERTIFICATE OF CAUSE OF DEATH

(For hospital in-patients, not to be used for stillbirths)

Mrs Ramvati, a 70-year-old obese female was admitted in the ICU with dyspnea and moderate retrosternal pain of 3 hours duration, which did not respond to nitroglycerin. There was a past history of noninsulin-dependent diabetes mellitus, hypertension and episodes of nonexertional chest pain, diagnosed as angina pectoris for 8 years. Over the next 72 hours, she developed a significant elevation of the MB isoenzyme of creatine phosphokinase, confirming an acute myocardial infarction. A Type II second-degree AV block developed, and a temporary pacemaker was put in place. She subsequently developed dyspnea with fluid retention and cardiomegaly on chest radiograph. On the 7th hospital day, during ambulation, she suddenly developed chest pain and increased dyspnea. An acute pulmonary embolism was suspected and intravenous heparin was started. The diagnosis of pulmonary embolism was confirmed by a ventilation/ perfusion scan as well as arterial blood gas measurements. One hour later, she became unresponsive and resuscitation efforts were unsuccessful. Fill up the death certificate in this case.

Name of Hospital ____________________

I hereby certify that the person whose particulars are given below died in the hospital Ward Number ________

____________________ on ____________________ at ____________________ AM/ PM.

NAME OF DECEASED ____________________

Sex	Age at Death			
1. Male 2. Female	If one year or more, age in years	If less than one year, age in months	If less than one month, age in days	If less than one day, age in hours

	Cause of death	Interval between onset and death (approx)
I. Immediate cause (State the disease, injury or complication, which caused death, not the mode of dying such as heart failure, asthenia, etc.)	a. Due to (or as a consequences of)	
Antecedent cause (Morbid conditions, if any giving rise to the above cause, stating underlying conditions last)	b. Due to (or as a consequences of) c.	
II. Other significant conditions contributing to the death but not related to the diseases or conditions causing it.		
Manner of Death: How did the injury occur? 1. Natural 2. Accident 3. Suicide 4. Homicide 5. Pending investigation		
If deceased was a female, was pregnancy the death associated with: 1. Yes 2. No If yes, was there a delivery? 1. Yes 2. No		

Name and signature of the Medical officer certifying the cause of death ____________________

Date of verification ____________________

EX. 6.2: MEDICAL CERTIFICATE OF CAUSE OF DEATH

(For hospital in-patients, not to be used for stillbirths)

Ritu Kumari, a 35-year-old gravida three, para two woman with gestational hypertension, reported to the emergency room at 36 weeks into her pregnancy. She had experienced 12 hours of abdominal cramping and vaginal bleeding with the passage of large clots. A presumptive diagnosis of abruptio placenta was made. She continued to bleed from her vagina as well as from phlebotomy sites, and she rapidly went into profound shock. No fetal heart sounds were audible. The patient was experiencing disseminated intravascular coagulation. Despite administration of blood and clotting factors, blood pressure could not be maintained. The mother and fetus both died 1 hour after admission. Fill up the death certificate in this case.

Name of Hospital ________________________________

I hereby certify that the person whose particulars are given below died in the hospital Ward Number __________

________________ on ________________ at ________________ AM/ PM.

NAME OF DECEASED ________________________________

Sex	Age at Death			
1. Male 2. Female	If one year or more, age in years	If less than one year, age in months	If less than one month, age in days	If less than one day, age in hours
		Cause of death		Interval between onset and death (approx)
I. Immediate cause (State the disease, injury or complication, which caused death, not the mode of dying such as heart failure, asthenia, etc.)		a. Due to (or as a consequences of)		
Antecedent cause (Morbid conditions, if any giving rise to the above cause, stating underlying conditions last)		b. Due to (or as a consequences of) c.		
II. Other significant conditions contributing to the death but not related to the diseases or conditions causing it.				
Manner of Death: How did the injury occur? 1. Natural	2. Accident	3. Suicide	4. Homicide	5. Pending investigation
If deceased was a female, was pregnancy the death associated with: If yes, was there a delivery?			1. Yes 1. Yes	2. No 2. No

Name and signature of the Medical officer certifying the cause of death ________________

Date of verification ________________

NOTES

NOTES

UNIT VII

Postmortem Examination

AUTOPSY REPORT FORMAT

Autopsy reports are medicolegal documents that not only report the anatomic findings of the postmortem examination but which also provide detailed clinic-pathologic correlations. It is important that the autopsy report should contain all the information necessary to support the cause of death statement.

Historical summary should include findings in scene investigations, history of incident, medical history, sign and symptoms before death, medical intervention, laboratory findings and imaging findings.

Identification features: Identifying marks and scars (including detailed descriptions of tattoos and healed surgical incisions), body weight and length, hair color and dentition are commonly recorded in unidentified bodies. Fingerprints are taken on separate sheet and attached with the report.

Presentation, clothing, personal effects and associated items: The documentation of how the body was received and the state of the remains before the examination is highly important. The clothing, jewellery and personal effects are to be documented (and photographed). Important areas be encircled on the clothing wherever possible and handed over to the police.

Evidence of medical intervention: All medical devices that were placed in the course of medical therapy should be documented. All tubes, catheters, puncture sites, bandages and other appliances that were placed in the patient are important and places iatrogenic artifacts into context.

Postmortem changes: Documentation of routine postmortem changes aids in interpretation of other autopsy findings. Rigor mortis, algor mortis, postmortem staining and decomposition changes etc. helps in establishing the postmortem interval and in interpretation of autopsy findings.

External examination: It requires detailed observations organized in a logical manner. Depending on the nature of the case, relevant negatives can be included throughout the report. Descriptions of body height, weight, nutrition, body symmetry, eyes, nose, ears, mouth, teeth, neck, chest, abdomen, genitalia, and extremities give the reader of the report a sense of the condition of the body at the time of the examination, and the quality of the detail gives credence to the overall accuracy and thoroughness of the report.

Internal examination: The internal examination is the central portion of the examination and deserves thoroughness and attention to detail that justifies the autopsy and the original goals of the examination. All internal organs should be inspected, weighed and described. All positive findings should have qualifiers [measurements, color or degree (e.g. mild, moderate, severe)] to give the reader a sense of the magnitude of the abnormality. If there is no disease or injury in the organ examined, it should be mentioned as *'healthy'*. Significant negatives should also be listed based on the peculiarities of the case. General protocol to follow is given in table.

Contd...

Protocol followed in internal examination

Body cavities (pleural, abdominal, pelvic)	• Organ arrangement • Presence or absence of fluids (straw/ turbid/ purulent/ hemorrhagic), effusions (large/ moderate/ small) and adhesions (dense/ scattered) • Appearance of viscera (degree of decomposition)
Head	• Configuration • Weight of brain • Hemorrhage, herniations, infection • Ventricular system • Pituitary • Scalp and skull • Meninges • Blood vessels • Orbital, nasal and aural cavities
Neck	• General appearance • Larynx and vocal cords • Thyroid cartilage • Trachea • Mouth, tongue and pharynx • Subcutaneous tissue and muscles • Hyoid bone
Respiratory system	• Lung weights • General appearance • Tracheobronchial tree • Parenchyma appearance, with details of diffuse or focal lesions • Diaphragm
Heart	• Weight • Coronary arteries • Valves (including circumferences, if abnormal) • Myocardium (including left and right ventricular wall thickness) • Hemopericardium (quantity) • Aorta and vena cava
GIT	• Esophagus • Stomach (wall condition, contents, quantity and smell) • Pancreas • Small and large intestine (perforation—site, obstruction—cause) • Rectum
Liver and biliary system	• Weight • Consistency • Color • Gallbladder and contents
Reticuloendothelial system	• Spleen weight • Thymus (if present) • Appearance of lymph nodes
Genitourinary tract	• Kidneys (weight and appearance) • Ureters • Bladder and urethra • Male/ female genital organs—contusion, abrasion in and around genital organs; in case of male—testes, and in case of female—condition of vagina and ovary, presence of foreign body in uterus, size, products of conception, semen or any other fluid
Musculoskeletal system	• General appearance of all bones, musculature and soft tissues

Histology and microscopic examination: Any tissue may be submitted for examination depending on the nature of the case.

Toxicology, laboratory, and ancillary procedure: The necessary tests should be done since such testing provides important information that is highly important to the final opinion of the cause of death.

EX. 7.1: BASICS OF POSTMORTEM EXAMINATION

A. **Definition**

B. **Types**

C. **Purpose/ Objectives**

D. **Types of skin incisions to open the body**

EX. 7.2A: POSTMORTEM INSTRUMENTS

Identify the instruments and mention its uses in autopsy.

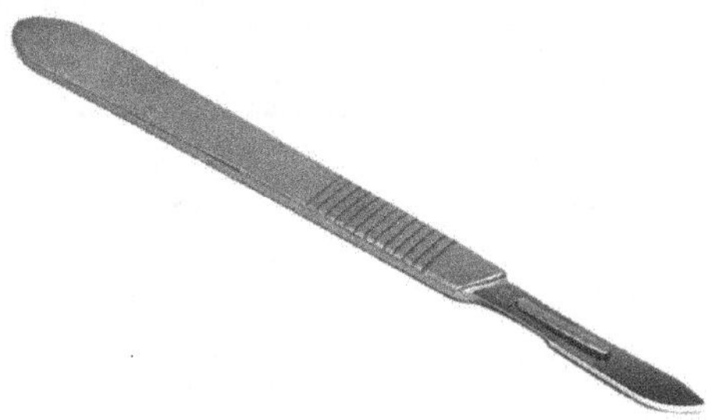	Name of the instrument: Uses:
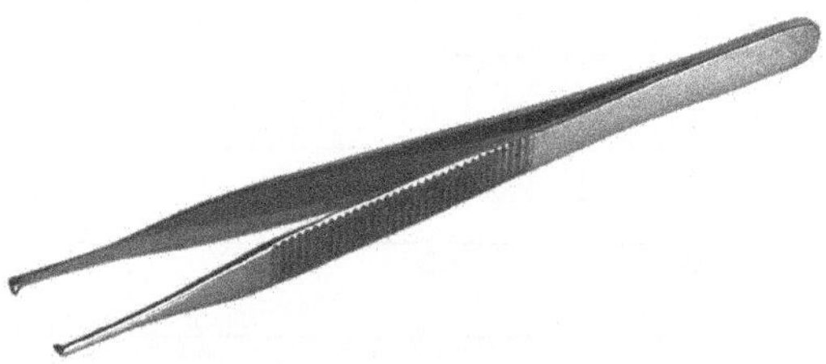	Name of the instrument: Uses:
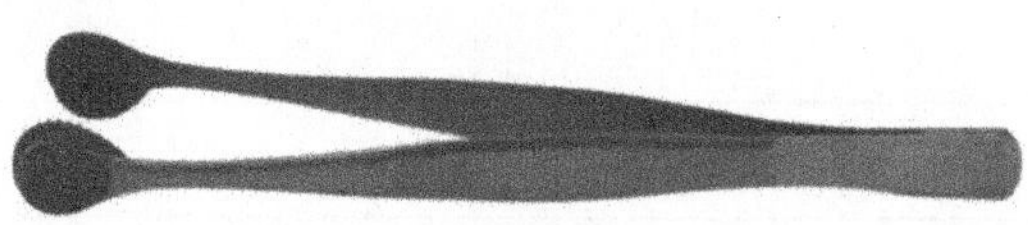	Name of the instrument: Uses:
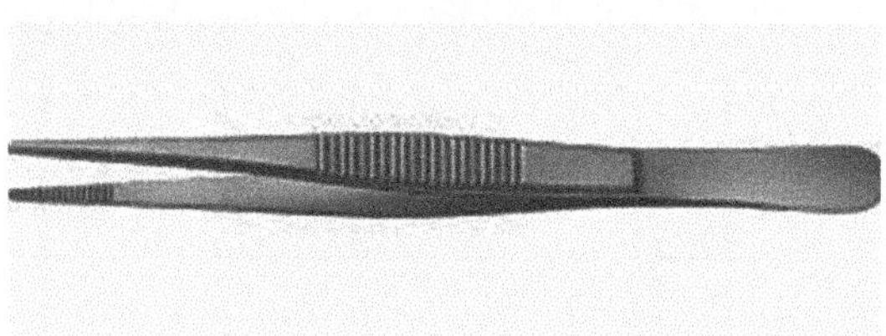	Name of the instrument: Uses:
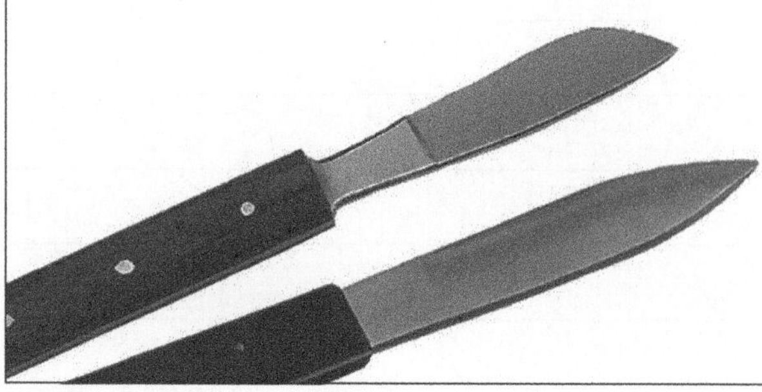	Name of the instrument: Uses:

EX. 7.2B: POSTMORTEM INSTRUMENTS

Identify the instruments and mention its uses in autopsy.

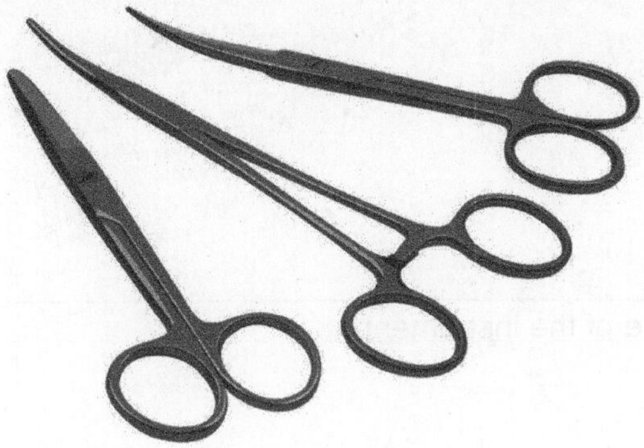	Name of the instrument: Uses:
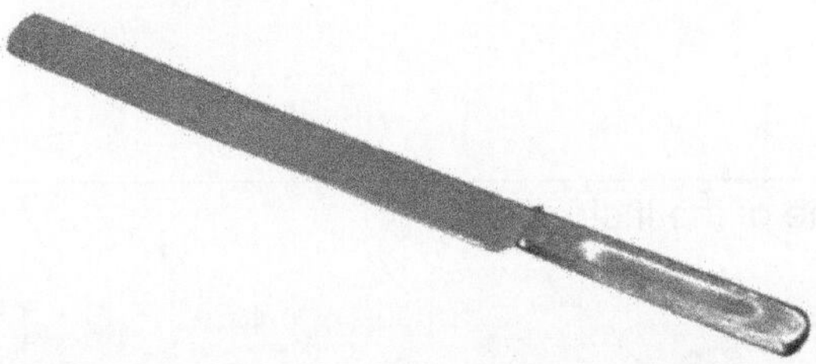	Name of the instrument: Uses:
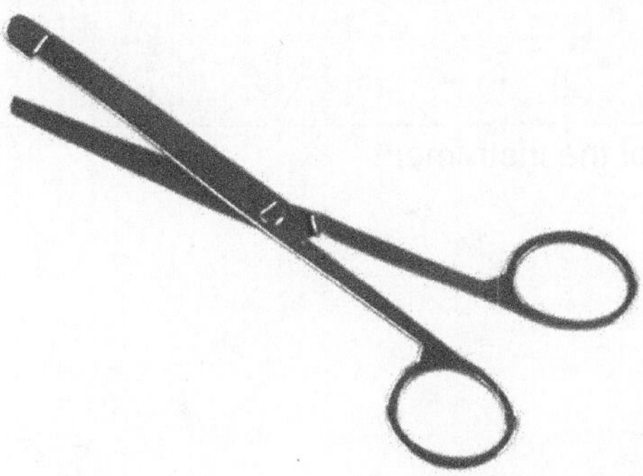	Name of the instrument: Uses:
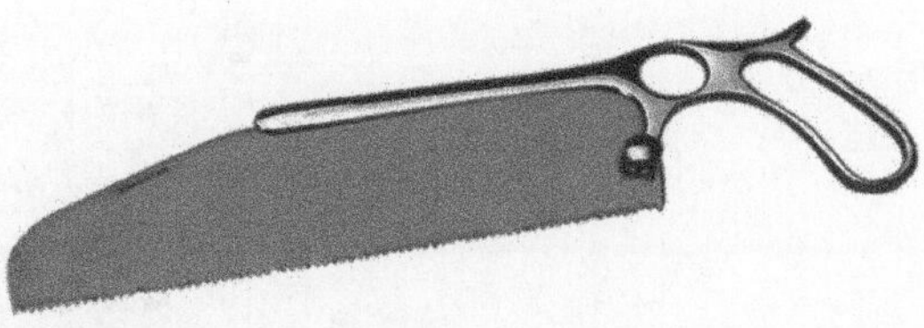	Name of the instrument: Uses:

EX. 7.2C: POSTMORTEM INSTRUMENTS

Identify the instruments and mention its uses in autopsy.

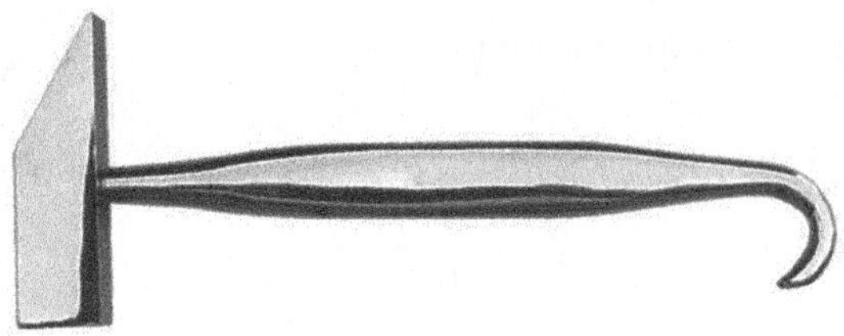	Name of the instrument: Uses:
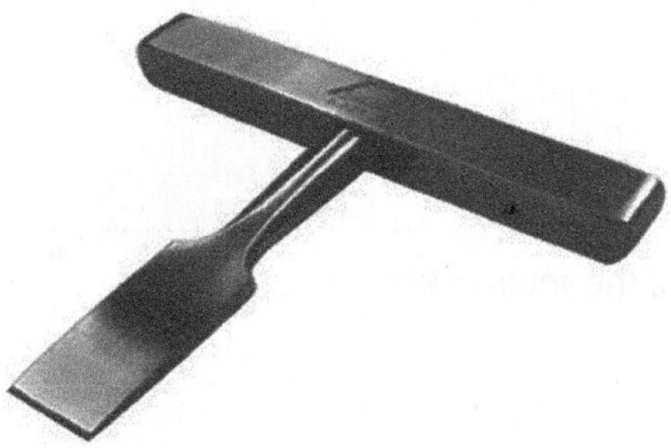	Name of the instrument: Uses:
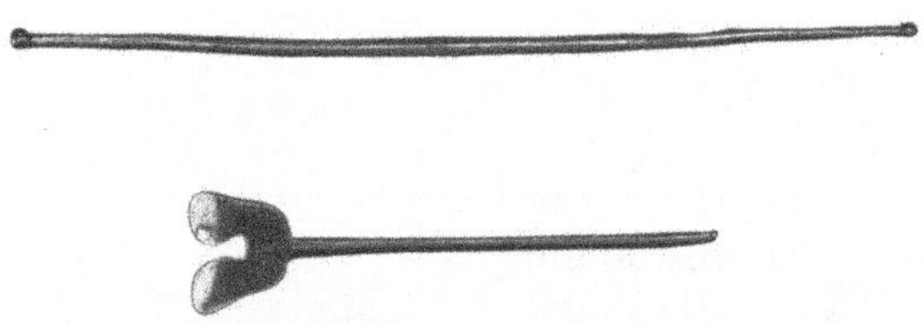	Name of the instrument: Uses:
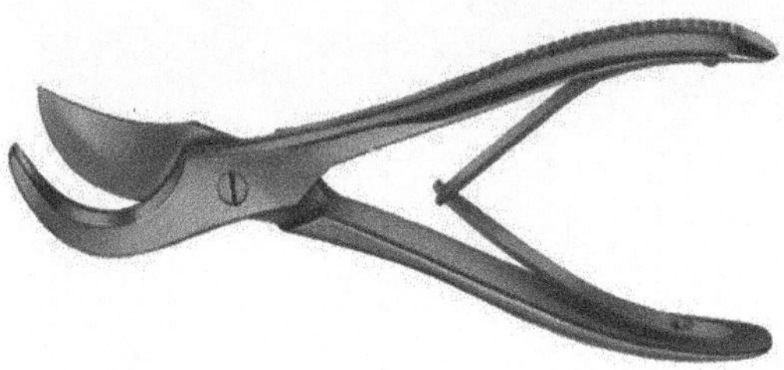	Name of the instrument: Uses:
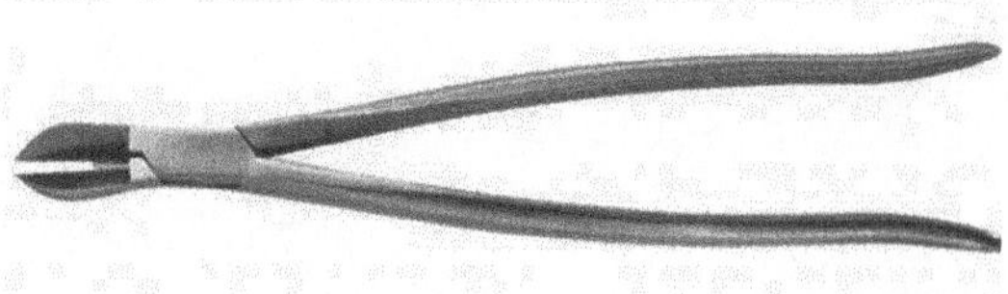	Name of the instrument: Uses:

EX. 7.2D: POSTMORTEM INSTRUMENTS

Identify the instruments and mention its uses in autopsy.

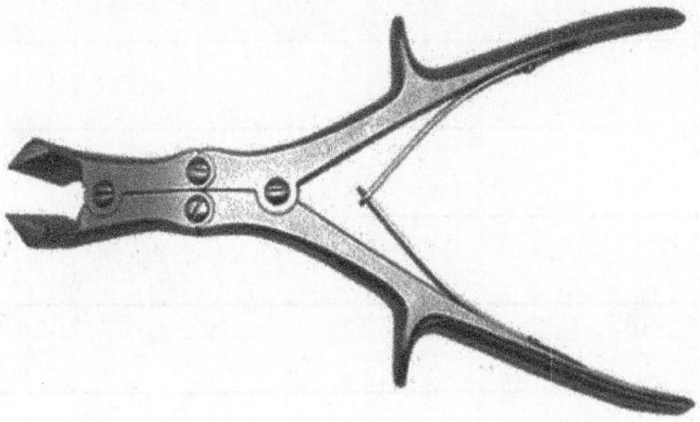	Name of the instrument: Uses:
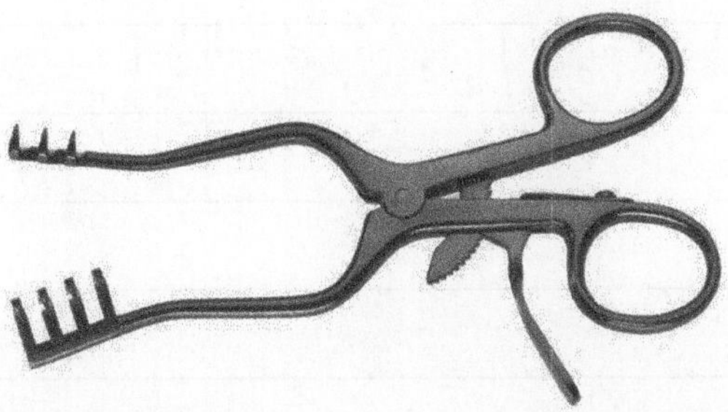	Name of the instrument: Uses:
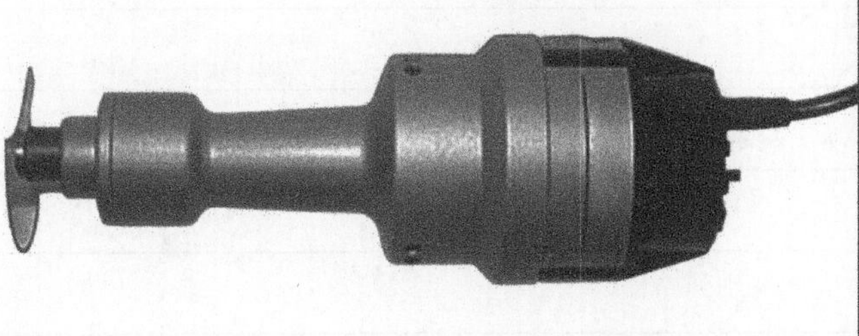	Name of the instrument: Uses:
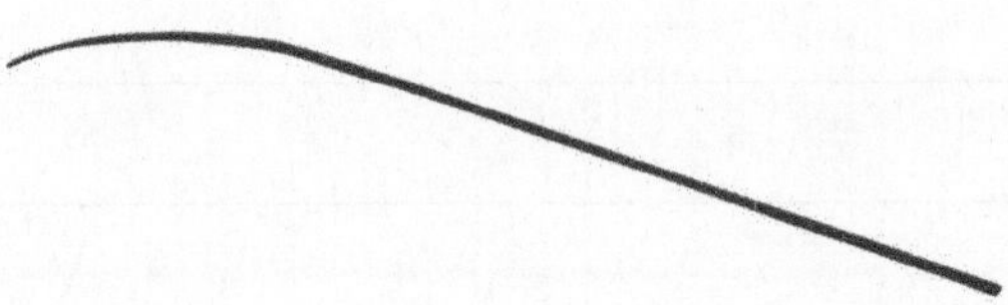	Name of the instrument: Uses:

EX. 7.3: PRESERVATION OF VISCERA

A. **Indications for preservation of viscera** ______

B. **Viscera preserved during autopsy (routinely)** ______

C. **Procedure of preservation of viscera (briefly)** ______

EX. 7.4: POSTMORTEM EXAMINATION OF FETUS

A female fetus of 49 cm crown heel length was brought to the mortuary with alleged history of killing of the baby after home delivery. But the mother claims it to be stillborn and is one month premature. Write a detailed autopsy report for the same.

Report No ______________________ Date ______________

Name ______________________________________ S/ D of ______________________

Address ____

Body identified by ______________________ Police personnel ______________________

Police Station ______________________________ District ______________________

A. EXTERNAL EXAMINATION

Clothings and wrappings (describe) ____

Length (cm)__________ Weight (gm) __________ Foot length (cm) __________

Circumference (cm): Head ______________ Chest ______________ Abdominal ______________

Sex (Male-M/ Female-F/ Ambiguous-A/ Undifferentiated-U) ☐

Hair	Scalp hair ________________ Lanugo hair: Present (mention areas) ______________/ Absent Eyebrows: Present/ Absent Eyelashes: Present/ Absent Adherent/ Separated
Vernix caseosa	Present (mention areas) ______________/ Absent
Skin	Normal/ Wrinkled/ Macerated/ Decomposed Surface injuries ____________________ Other (describe) ____________
Head	Normal/ Hydrocephalic/ Scalp defects/ Anencephalic/ Abnormal skull shape/ Collapsed/ Molding Trauma ________________________ Other (describe) ____________
Eyes	Normal/ Close together/ Far apart/ Straight/ Up slanting/ Down slanting/ Abnormally small/ Abnormally large/ Epicanthus Other (describe) __________ Conjunctiva ________________
Nose	Normal/ Other (describe) __________________________ Injuries ____
Mouth	Normal/ Cleft palate/ Cleft lip/ Large tongue/ Small chin Injuries ________________ Other (describe) ____________

Ears	Normal/ Lowset/ Tags/ Pits/ Symmetric Level of crest with lateral canthus ___________	Plasticity ________________ Other (describe) ___________
Neck	Normal/ Excess skin/ Cystic mass Injuries ______________________________	Other (describe) _____________
Chest	Normal/ Asymmetric/ Small/ Other __________	
Abdomen	Normal/ Distended/ Omphalocele/ Gastroschisis/ Hernia/ 3-vessel cord Other ____	
Back	Normal/ Spina bifida (defect level _____)/ Scoliosis/ Kyphosis Other (describe) ____	
Limbs	Length (Normal/ short/ long) Form (Normal/ symmetric/ missing parts)	Position (Normal/ abnormal)
Arms Right Left Legs Right Left		
Hands Right Left	 Fingers ( ), Webbing/ Syndactyly/ Transverse crease Fingers ( ), Webbing/ Syndactyly/ Transverse crease	 Other ___________ Other ___________
Feet Right Left	 Toes ( ), Webbing/ Wide space between toes 1–2 Toes ( ), Webbing/ Wide space between toes 1–2	 Other ___________ Other ___________
Nails	Normal/ Small (which ones?) ______________ Level with fingers ________________	Other ___________
Genitalia	Normal/ Imperforate anus Ambiguous genitalia (describe) ________________________	
Male	Hypospadias/ Chordee/ Undescended testes (right/ left) ________________ Other (describe) ____________	
Female	Normal/ Abnormal urethral opening Clitromegaly: Yes/ No Other (describe) ____________	

Injuries (any other/ burns/ fracture): ____

____

____

____

____

Any other mass (Yes/ No), if yes, describe ______________________________________

B. INTERNAL EXAMINATION

Head and Neck

Scalp:

Cephalhematoma and caput succedaneum:

Fontanelles:

Skull:

Meninges:

Brain:

Neck:

Thorax

Level of diaphragm:

Thymus:

Pleura:

Lungs: Wt (gm) Right ________ Left ________ Volume ________ Margins ________

Consistency: Crepitant/ Noncrepitant Color: Reddish brown/ Salmon-pink

Sectioning: Frothless blood/ Frothy blood

Hydrostatic test:

Heart: Wt (gm) ________

Condition of valves:

Foramen ovale:

Abdomen

Stomach (contents):

Intestines (meconium presence and site):

Liver: Size (cm) ________ Wt (gm) ________ Consistency: Soft/ Firm/ Hard

Gallbladder: Absent/ Present

Spleen: Size (cm) ________ Wt (gm) ________ Consistency: Soft/ Firm/ Hard

Kidneys: Size (cm) Right ________ Left ________

Wt (gm) Right ________ Left ________

Ureters:

Urinary bladder:

OSSIFICATION CENTERS *(Tick '√')*

☐ Calcaneum ☐ Sternum ☐ Talus

☐ Lower end of femur ☐ Upper end of tibia

UMBILICAL CORD

Umbilical cord length (cm) ___________ Normal/ Abnormal

Umbilical vessels ____________________ Condition of cord _______________________

PLACENTA EXAMINATION

Weight (gm) ___________________ Diameter (cm) ______________________

Morphology: Normal/ Abnormal

Cord insertion: Normal/ Abnormal Infarct Yes/ No

Chorionicity of multiple pregnancy ___________________________

Membrane culture Negative/ Positive

Histopathology Done/ Not done Suggestive of syphilis Yes/ No

PRESERVATION OF SAMPLES (for DNA, blood grouping and toxicological screening)

1. ____
2. ____
3. ____

OPINION

____

____

____

Place __________

Date __________

Signature of the Doctor

Name, Designation and Seal

Received PM report No. ____________________ along with ___________________ number of envelopes and ________________________ number of samples and sample seal.

Name________________________ P.C.No.________________________ P.S.________________

Signature and date

EX. 7.5.1: POSTMORTEM REPORT

Department of Forensic Medicine and Toxicology

____

P.M. Report No. _______________ C.R. No. ____________
(in case of hospital admission)

Date and time of receipt of body ____________________

Date and time of receipt of inquest papers ______________

Date and time of commencement of autopsy ____________________

Time of completion of autopsy _________ AM/PM

In case of hospital deaths (particular as per hospital records)

Date and time of admission _______________ Date and time of death _______________

Body brought by (Name, signature and rank/ number of police official) _________________________

__________________________________ Police Station _________________________

Identified by (Name and addresses of relatives/ persons acquainted along with their signature)

1. ____
2. ____

History (all events prior to death) ____

____

____

Information furnished by: ____________________________

Particulars of Deceased

Name ____________________________ Father's/ Husband's Name _________________________

Sex ____________________ Age _________________ Race/ Religion ________________________

Address ____

Identifications marks (if body is unidentified)

1. ____
2. ____

Height __________ cm Weight ____________ kg

Circumcision: Yes/ No Beard, mustache __________________

.... Signature of the doctor

SCHEDULE OF OBSERVATIONS

A. General	
Body	Entire and intact/ Mutilated and in pieces
Clothings	
Medical intervention (if any)	
Built	Well/ Moderate/ Poor/ Emaciated
Nourishment/ Physique	Lean/ Medium/ Obese
Scars/ Tattoos/ Bedsores (if present)	
Skin	Pallor/ Jaundiced/ Pink/ Cyanosis
Facial appearance	Pale/ Normal/ Livid/ Cyanosed
Eyes Cornea Pupils Conjunctivae	Closed/ Half open/ Open Clear/ Hazy/ Opaque Arcus senilis: Absent/ Developing/ Fully developed Constricted/ Dilated Regular/ Irregular Pale/ Normal/ Congested/ Jaundiced/ Hemorrhagic
Nostrils	
Ears	
Mouth	
Teeth	
Tongue	
Oral cavity	
Circum-oral regions Lips Inner aspects of lips Frenulum	 Pale/ Cyanosed Intact/ Torn
Orifice Urethral Anal Vaginal (in females)	
Condition of limbs	
Rigor mortis	Developing/ Fully developed/ Passing off Mild/ Strong
Postmortem staining	Fixed/ Not fixed Areas present____________
Decomposition changes Skin Face/ abdomen/ scrotum Foul smell Maggots	 Color changes of putrefaction/ Marbling/ Skin slippage Bloated/ Not bloated Present/ Absent Present/ Absent
Any other findings	

....................Signature of the doctor

B. External Injuries
(Mention type, shape, length × breadth × depth of each injury and its relation to important body landmark. Indicate which injuries are fresh and which are old and their duration)

C. Internal Examination	
Head Scalp Skull Brain	
Neck	
Chest Ribs/ sternum/ chest wall Pleural cavities Lungs Right Left Pericardium Heart Coronaries Large blood vessels	
Abdomen Peritoneum Stomach and its contents Small intestines its contents Large intestines and its contents Liver Gallbladder Spleen Pancreas Kidneys and ureters Urinary bladder Pelvic cavity	

* Injuries are to be given in serial number and mark them on the diagrams attached. In stab injuries, mention angles, margins and direction inside the body. In firearms injuries, mention direction and effects of fire.

……………………Signature of the doctor

Genital organs	
Spinal columns and spinal cord (opened where indicated)	

OPINION

a. Probable time since death (keeping all factors including observations at inquest)

   i. Between injury and death ____________________

   ii. Between death and postmortem examination ____________________

b. Cause and manner of death. The cause of death to the best of my knowledge and belief is:

   i. Immediate cause ____________________

   ii. Due to ____________________

   iii. Which of the injuries are antemortem/ postmortem and duration if antemortem? ____________________

   ____

   iv. Manner of causation of injuries (if possible) ____________________

   v. Whether injuries (individually or collectively) are sufficient to cause death in ordinary course of nature or not? ____________________

c. Any other ____________________

Specimens collected and preserved *(Tick '√')*

- ☐ Viscera (1. Stomach and small intestines with its contents, 2. Part of liver, half of each kidneys, spleen 3. Blood 4. Urine 5. Preservative used for sample 1 and 2, 6. Preservative used for sample 3 and 4)
- ☐ Sample of blood in gauze piece (dried)
- ☐ Clothes (air dried)
- ☐ Photographs/ Video CD in case of custody deaths/ Fingerprints
- ☐ Foreign body (like bullet, ligature)
- ☐ Slides from vagina or any other material ____________________
- ☐ Organs for histopathological examination

Place __________

____

Signature of the Doctor

Name (block letters), Designation and Seal

Received PM report No. ____________________ in original/copy along with body diagram and

____________________ inquest papers (mention total number and initial them all).

(Viscera or any other specimen, if preserved is handed over to the police immediately after autopsy)

Name ____________________ P.C. No. ____________________ P.S. ____________________

____

Signature and date

Date ____________ **PMR No.** ____________

Right Side | Front | Back | Left Side

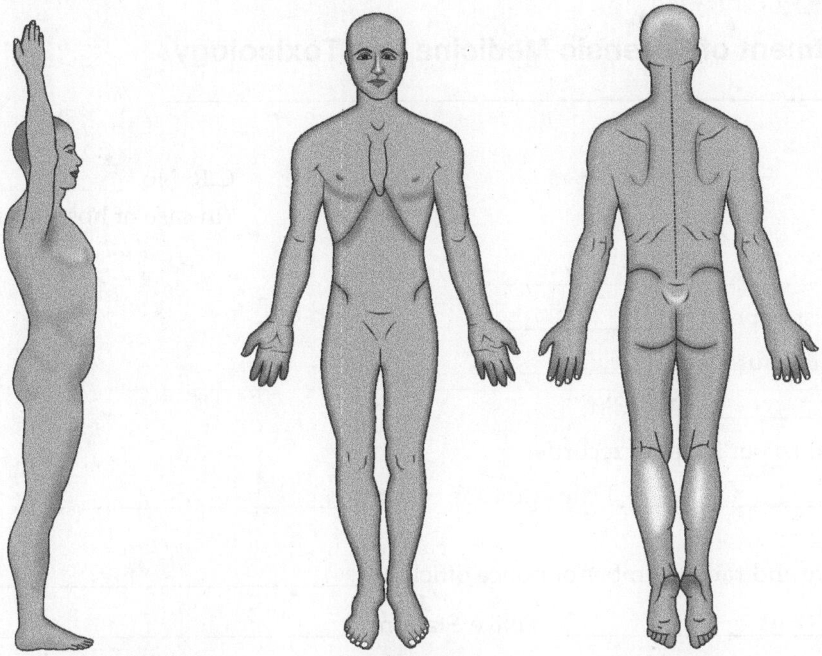

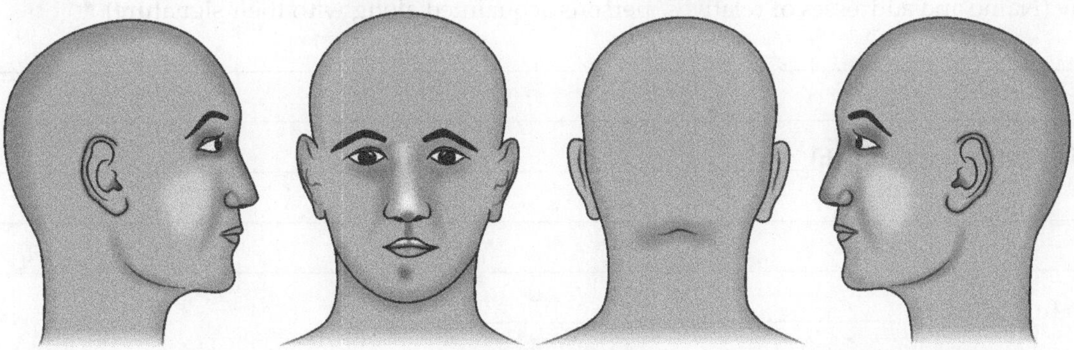

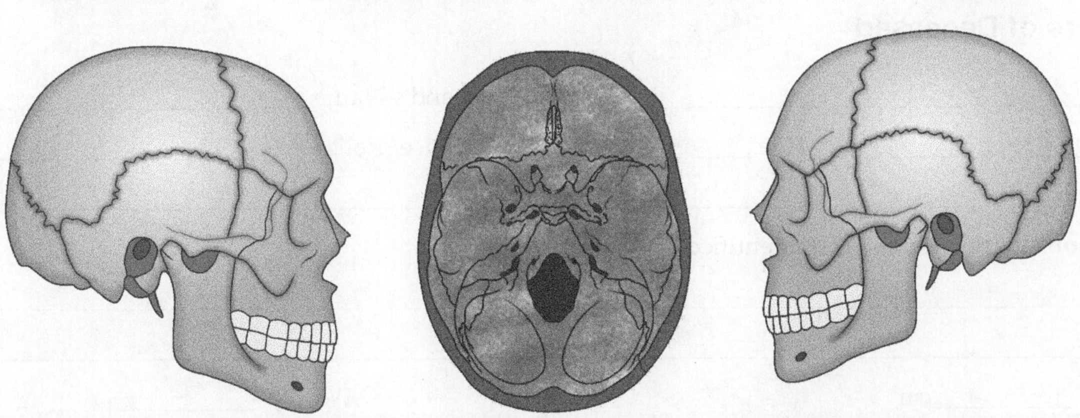

Signature of the Doctor
Name, Designation and Seal

EX. 7.5.2: POSTMORTEM REPORT

Department of Forensic Medicine and Toxicology

____

P.M. Report No. ________________

C.R. No. ________________
(in case of hospital admission)

Date and time of receipt of body ________________________

Date and time of receipt of inquest papers ________________

Date and time of commencement of autopsy ______________________

Time of completion of autopsy __________ AM/PM

In case of hospital deaths (particular as per hospital records)

Date and time of admission __________________ Date and time of death __________________

Body brought by (Name, signature and rank/ number of police official) ____________________________________

____ Police Station ___________________________________

Identified by (Name and addresses of relatives/ persons acquainted along with their signature)

1. ____
2. ____

History (all events prior to death) ____

____

____

Information furnished by: ____________________________________

Particulars of Deceased

Name _____________________________________ Father's/ Husband's Name ________________________________

Sex __________________________ Age ______________________ Race/ Religion ______________________________

Address ____

Identifications marks (if body is unidentified)

1. ____
2. ____

Height ______________ cm Weight ________________ kg

Circumcision: Yes/ No Beard, mustache ____________________

.... Signature of the doctor

SCHEDULE OF OBSERVATIONS

A. General	
Body	Entire and intact/ Mutilated and in pieces
Clothings	
Medical intervention (if any)	
Built	Well/ Moderate/ Poor/ Emaciated
Nourishment/ Physique	Lean/ Medium/ Obese
Scars/ Tattoos/ Bedsores (if present)	
Skin	Pallor/ Jaundiced/ Pink/ Cyanosis
Facial appearance	Pale/ Normal/ Livid/ Cyanosed
Eyes Cornea Pupils Conjunctivae	Closed/ Half open/ Open Clear/ Hazy/ Opaque Arcus senilis: Absent/ Developing/ Fully developed Constricted/ Dilated Regular/ Irregular Pale/ Normal/ Congested/ Jaundiced/ Hemorrhagic
Nostrils	
Ears	
Mouth	
Teeth	
Tongue	
Oral cavity	
Circum-oral regions Lips Inner aspects of lips Frenulum	 Pale/ Cyanosed Intact/ Torn
Orifice Urethral Anal Vaginal (in females)	
Condition of limbs	
Rigor mortis	Developing/ Fully developed/ Passing off Mild/ Strong
Postmortem staining	Fixed/ Not fixed Areas present________________
Decomposition changes Skin Face/ abdomen/ scrotum Foul smell Maggots	 Color changes of putrefaction/ Marbling/ Skin slippage Bloated/ Not bloated Present/ Absent Present/ Absent
Any other findings	

……………………Signature of doctor

B. External Injuries
(Mention type, shape, length × breadth × depth of each injury and its relation to important body landmark. Indicate which injuries are fresh and which are old and their duration)

C. Internal Examination	
Head Scalp Skull Brain	
Neck	
Chest Ribs/ sternum/ chest wall Pleural cavities Lungs Right Left Pericardium Heart Coronaries Large blood vessels	
Abdomen Peritoneum Stomach and its contents Small intestines its contents Large intestines and its contents Liver Gallbladder Spleen Pancreas Kidneys and ureters Urinary bladder Pelvic cavity	

* Injuries are to be given in serial number and mark them on the diagrams attached. In stab injuries, mention angles, margins and direction inside the body. In firearms injuries, mention direction and effects of fire.

.....................Signature of the doctor

Genital organs	
Spinal columns and spinal cord (opened where indicated)	

OPINION

a. Probable time since death (keeping all factors including observations at inquest)

   i. Between injury and death ______

   ii. Between death and postmortem examination ______

b. Cause and manner of death. The cause of death to the best of my knowledge and belief is:

   i. Immediate cause ______

   ii. Due to ______

   iii. Which of the injuries are antemortem/ postmortem and duration if antemortem? ______

   ______

   iv. Manner of causation of injuries (if possible) ______

   v. Whether injuries (individually or collectively) are sufficient to cause death in ordinary course of nature or not? ______

c. Any other ______

Specimens collected and preserved *(Tick '√')*

☐ Viscera (1. Stomach and small intestines with its contents, 2. Part of liver, half of each kidneys, spleen 3. Blood 4. Urine 5. Preservative used for sample 1 and 2, 6. Preservative used for sample 3 and 4)
☐ Sample of blood in gauze piece (dried)
☐ Clothes (air dried)
☐ Photographs/ Video CD in case of custody deaths/ Fingerprints
☐ Foreign body (like bullet, ligature)
☐ Slides from vagina or any other material ______
☐ Organs for histopathological examination

Place ______

______
Signature of the Doctor
Name (block letters), Designation and Seal

Received PM report No. ______ in original/copy along with body diagram and ______ inquest papers (mention total number and initial them all).

(Viscera or any other specimen, if preserved is handed over to the police immediately after autopsy)

Name ______ P.C. No. ______ P.S. ______

______
Signature and date

Date ______________ PMR No. ______________

Right Side Front Back Left Side

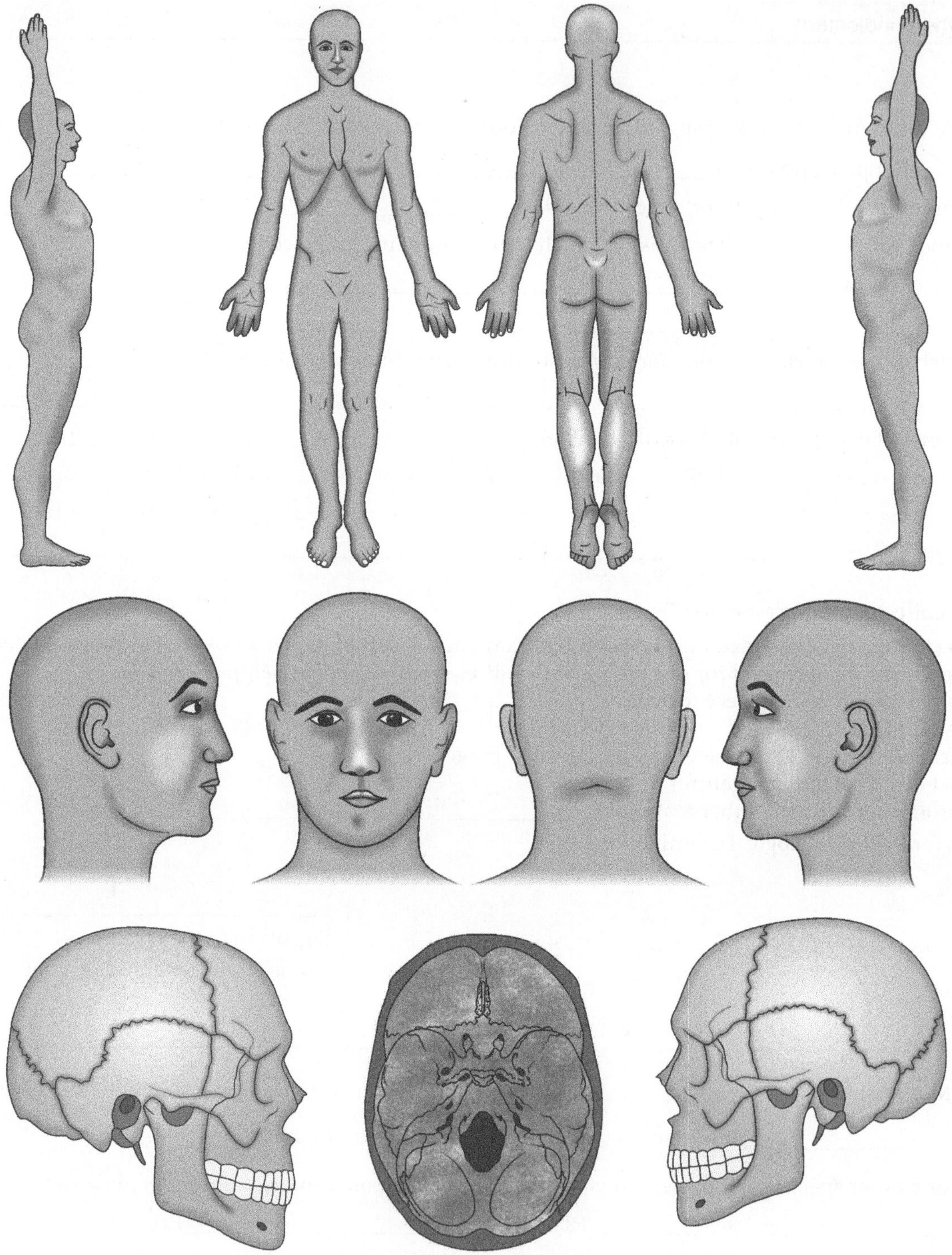

Signature of the Doctor
Name, Designation and Seal

EX. 7.5.3: POSTMORTEM REPORT

Department of Forensic Medicine and Toxicology

____

P.M. Report No. ________________ C.R. No. ________________
(in case of hospital admission)

Date and time of receipt of body ______________________
Date and time of receipt of inquest papers _______________
Date and time of commencement of autopsy ______________________
Time of completion of autopsy __________ AM/PM
In case of hospital deaths (particular as per hospital records)
Date and time of admission ________________ Date and time of death ________________

Body brought by (Name, signature and rank/ number of police official) ________________
________________________________ Police Station ________________

Identified by (Name and addresses of relatives/ persons acquainted along with their signature)

1. ________________________________
2. ________________________________

History (all events prior to death) ________________________________
____
____

Information furnished by: ________________________

Particulars of Deceased

Name ________________________ Father's/ Husband's Name ________________
Sex ________________ Age ________________ Race/ Religion ________________
Address ________________________________

Identifications marks (if body is unidentified)

1. ________________________________
2. ________________________________

Height ____________ cm Weight ____________ kg
Circumcision: Yes/ No Beard, mustache ________________

.... Signature of the doctor

SCHEDULE OF OBSERVATIONS

A. General	
Body	Entire and intact/ Mutilated and in pieces
Clothings	
Medical intervention (if any)	
Built	Well/ Moderate/ Poor/ Emaciated
Nourishment/ Physique	Lean/ Medium/ Obese
Scars/ Tattoos/ Bedsores (if present)	
Skin	Pallor/ Jaundiced/ Pink/ Cyanosis
Facial appearance	Pale/ Normal/ Livid/ Cyanosed
Eyes Cornea Pupils Conjunctivae	Closed/ Half open/ Open Clear/ Hazy/ Opaque Arcus senilis: Absent/ Developing/ Fully developed Constricted/ Dilated Regular/ Irregular Pale/ Normal/ Congested/ Jaundiced/ Hemorrhagic
Nostrils	
Ears	
Mouth	
Teeth	
Tongue	
Oral cavity	
Circum-oral regions Lips Inner aspects of lips Frenulum	 Pale/ Cyanosed Intact/ Torn
Orifice Urethral Anal Vaginal (in females)	
Condition of limbs	
Rigor mortis	Developing/ Fully developed/ Passing off Mild/ Strong
Postmortem staining	Fixed/ Not fixed Areas present__________________
Decomposition changes Skin Face/ abdomen/ scrotum Foul smell Maggots	 Color changes of putrefaction/ Marbling/ Skin slippage Bloated/ Not bloated Present/ Absent Present/ Absent
Any other findings	

.... Signature of doctor

B. External Injuries
(Mention type, shape, length × breadth × depth of each injury and its relation to important body landmark. Indicate which injuries are fresh and which are old and their duration)

C. Internal Examination	
Head Scalp Skull Brain	
Neck	
Chest Ribs/ sternum/ chest wall Pleural cavities Lungs Right Left Pericardium Heart Coronaries Large blood vessels	
Abdomen Peritoneum Stomach and its contents Small intestines its contents Large intestines and its contents Liver Gallbladder Spleen Pancreas Kidneys and ureters Urinary bladder Pelvic cavity	

* Injuries are to be given in serial number and mark them on the diagrams attached. In stab injuries, mention angles, margins and direction inside the body. In firearms injuries, mention direction and effects of fire.

……………………Signature of the doctor

Genital organs	
Spinal columns and spinal cord (opened where indicated)	

OPINION

a. Probable time since death (keeping all factors including observations at inquest)
   i. Between injury and death ____________
   ii. Between death and postmortem examination ____________

b. Cause and manner of death. The cause of death to the best of my knowledge and belief is:
   i. Immediate cause ____________
   ii. Due to ____________
   iii. Which of the injuries are antemortem/ postmortem and duration if antemortem? ____________
   ____
   iv. Manner of causation of injuries (if possible) ____________
   v. Whether injuries (individually or collectively) are sufficient to cause death in ordinary course of nature or not? ____________

c. Any other ____________

Specimens collected and preserved *(Tick '√')*

- ☐ Viscera (1. Stomach and small intestines with its contents, 2. Part of liver, half of each kidneys, spleen 3. Blood 4. Urine 5. Preservative used for sample 1 and 2, 6. Preservative used for sample 3 and 4)
- ☐ Sample of blood in gauze piece (dried)
- ☐ Clothes (air dried)
- ☐ Photographs/ Video CD in case of custody deaths/ Fingerprints
- ☐ Foreign body (like bullet, ligature)
- ☐ Slides from vagina or any other material ____________
- ☐ Organs for histopathological examination

Place ________

____
Signature of the Doctor
Name (block letters), Designation and Seal

Received PM report No. ____________ in original/copy along with body diagram and ____________ inquest papers (mention total number and initial them all).

(Viscera or any other specimen, if preserved is handed over to the police immediately after autopsy)

Name ____________ P.C. No. ____________ P.S. ____________

____
Signature and date

Date ______________ **PMR No.** ______________

Right Side Front Back Left Side

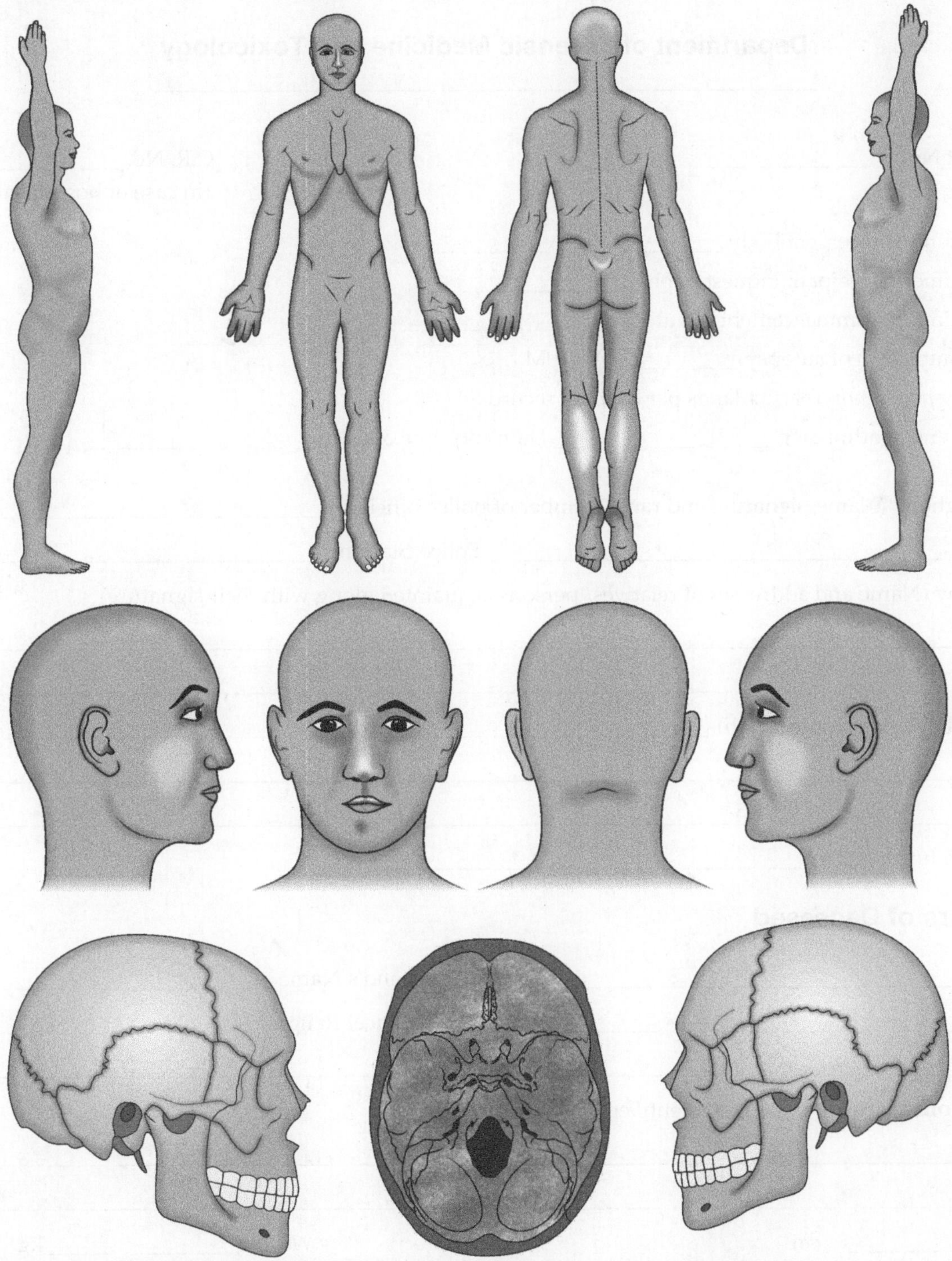

____

Signature of the Doctor
Name, Designation and Seal

EX. 7.5.4: POSTMORTEM REPORT

Department of Forensic Medicine and Toxicology

____

P.M. Report No. ______________ C.R. No. ______________
(in case of hospital admission)

Date and time of receipt of body ______________

Date and time of receipt of inquest papers ______________

Date and time of commencement of autopsy ______________

Time of completion of autopsy __________ AM/PM

In case of hospital deaths (particular as per hospital records)

Date and time of admission ______________ Date and time of death ______________

Body brought by (Name, signature and rank/ number of police official) ______________

______________ Police Station ______________

Identified by (Name and addresses of relatives/ persons acquainted along with their signature)

1. ______________
2. ______________

History (all events prior to death) ______________

____

____

Information furnished by: ______________

Particulars of Deceased

Name ______________ Father's/ Husband's Name ______________

Sex ______________ Age ______________ Race/ Religion ______________

Address ______________

Identifications marks (if body is unidentified)

1. ______________
2. ______________

Height ______________ cm Weight ______________ kg

Circumcision: Yes/ No Beard, mustache ______________

.... Signature of the doctor

SCHEDULE OF OBSERVATIONS

A. General	
Body	Entire and intact/ Mutilated and in pieces
Clothings	
Medical intervention (if any)	
Built	Well/ Moderate/ Poor/ Emaciated
Nourishment/ Physique	Lean/ Medium/ Obese
Scars/ Tattoos/ Bedsores (if present)	
Skin	Pallor/ Jaundiced/ Pink/ Cyanosis
Facial appearance	Pale/ Normal/ Livid/ Cyanosed
Eyes Cornea Pupils Conjunctivae	Closed/ Half open/ Open Clear/ Hazy/ Opaque Arcus senilis: Absent/ Developing/ Fully developed Constricted/ Dilated Regular/ Irregular Pale/ Normal/ Congested/ Jaundiced/ Hemorrhagic
Nostrils	
Ears	
Mouth	
Teeth	
Tongue	
Oral cavity	
Circum-oral regions Lips Inner aspects of lips Frenulum	 Pale/ Cyanosed Intact/ Torn
Orifice Urethral Anal Vaginal (in females)	
Condition of limbs	
Rigor mortis	Developing/ Fully developed/ Passing off Mild/ Strong
Postmortem staining	Fixed/ Not fixed Areas present________________________
Decomposition changes Skin Face/ abdomen/ scrotum Foul smell Maggots	 Color changes of putrefaction/ Marbling/ Skin slippage Bloated/ Not bloated Present/ Absent Present/ Absent
Any other findings	

.... Signature of doctor

B. External Injuries
(Mention type, shape, length × breadth × depth of each injury and its relation to important body landmark. Indicate which injuries are fresh and which are old and their duration)

C. Internal Examination	
Head Scalp Skull Brain	
Neck	
Chest Ribs/ sternum/ chest wall Pleural cavities Lungs Right Left Pericardium Heart Coronaries Large blood vessels	
Abdomen Peritoneum Stomach and its contents Small intestines its contents Large intestines and its contents Liver Gallbladder Spleen Pancreas Kidneys and ureters Urinary bladder Pelvic cavity	

* Injuries are to be given in serial number and mark them on the diagrams attached. In stab injuries, mention angles, margins and direction inside the body. In firearms injuries, mention direction and effects of fire.

……………………Signature of the doctor

Genital organs	
Spinal columns and spinal cord (opened where indicated)	

OPINION

a. Probable time since death (keeping all factors including observations at inquest)

  i. Between injury and death ______

  ii. Between death and postmortem examination ______

b. Cause and manner of death. The cause of death to the best of my knowledge and belief is:

  i. Immediate cause ______

  ii. Due to ______

  iii. Which of the injuries are antemortem/ postmortem and duration if antemortem? ______

  ______

  iv. Manner of causation of injuries (if possible) ______

  v. Whether injuries (individually or collectively) are sufficient to cause death in ordinary course of nature or not? ______

c. Any other ______

Specimens collected and preserved *(Tick '√')*

- ☐ Viscera (1. Stomach and small intestines with its contents, 2. Part of liver, half of each kidneys, spleen 3. Blood 4. Urine 5. Preservative used for sample 1 and 2, 6. Preservative used for sample 3 and 4)
- ☐ Sample of blood in gauze piece (dried)
- ☐ Clothes (air dried)
- ☐ Photographs/ Video CD in case of custody deaths/ Fingerprints
- ☐ Foreign body (like bullet, ligature)
- ☐ Slides from vagina or any other material ______
- ☐ Organs for histopathological examination

______

Place ______

Signature of the Doctor
Name (block letters), Designation and Seal

Received PM report No. ______ in original/copy along with body diagram and ______ inquest papers (mention total number and initial them all).

(Viscera or any other specimen, if preserved is handed over to the police immediately after autopsy)

Name ______ P.C. No. ______ P.S. ______

______

Signature and date

Date ________________ **PMR No.** ________________

Right Side Front Back Left Side

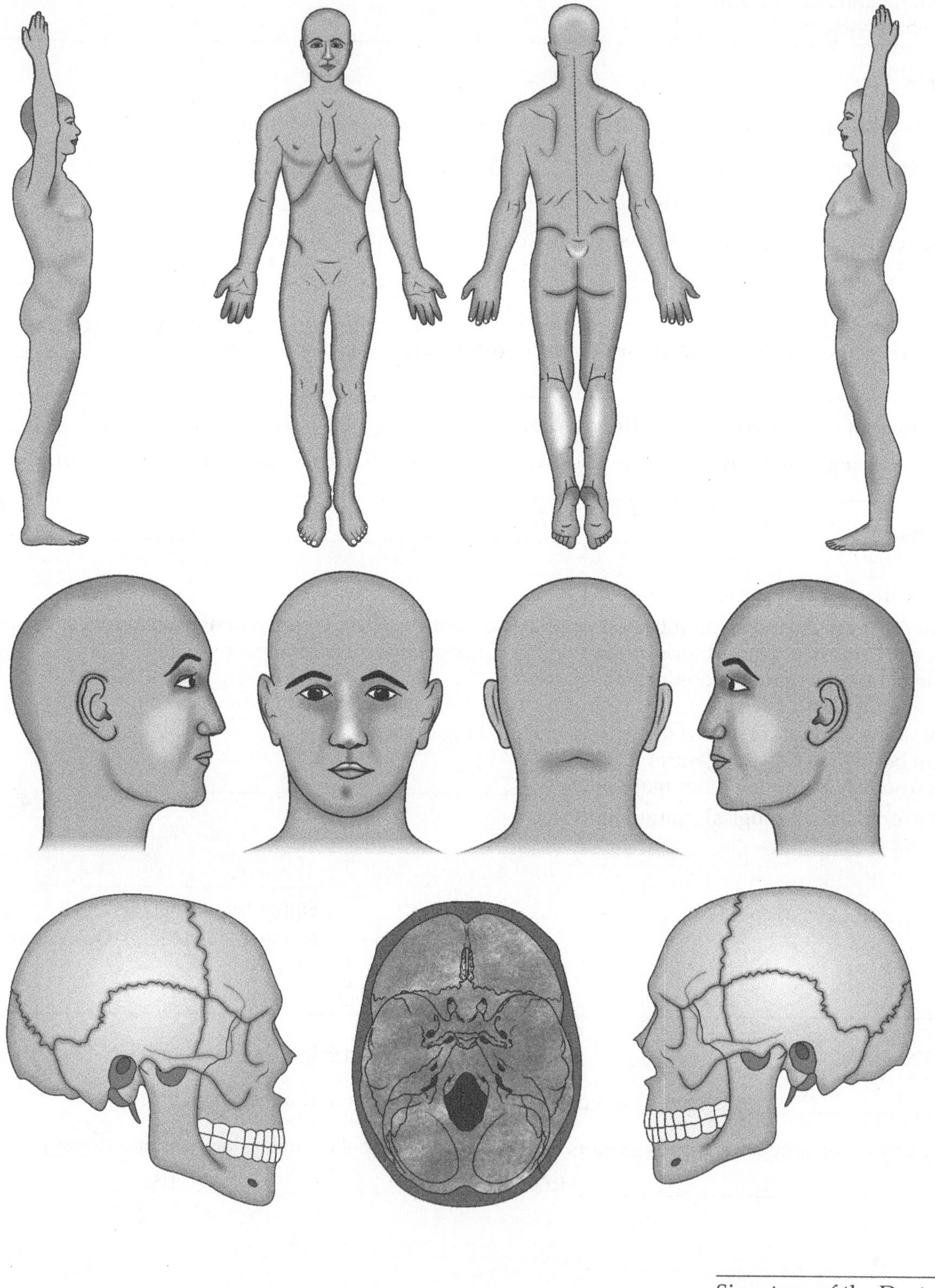

____

Signature of the Doctor
Name, Designation and Seal

EX. 7.5.5: POSTMORTEM REPORT

Department of Forensic Medicine and Toxicology

____

P.M. Report No. ______________ C.R. No. ______________
(in case of hospital admission)

Date and time of receipt of body ______________________

Date and time of receipt of inquest papers _______________

Date and time of commencement of autopsy _______________

Time of completion of autopsy __________ AM/PM

In case of hospital deaths (particular as per hospital records)

Date and time of admission ______________ Date and time of death ______________

Body brought by (Name, signature and rank/ number of police official) ______________________

______________________ Police Station ______________________

Identified by (Name and addresses of relatives/ persons acquainted along with their signature)

1. ____

2. ____

History (all events prior to death) ____

____

____

Information furnished by: ______________________

Particulars of Deceased

Name ______________________ Father's/ Husband's Name ______________________

Sex ______________ Age ______________ Race/ Religion ______________

Address ____

Identifications marks (if body is unidentified)

1. ____

2. ____

Height __________ cm Weight __________ kg

Circumcision: Yes/ No Beard, mustache ______________

.... Signature of the doctor

SCHEDULE OF OBSERVATIONS

A. General	
Body	Entire and intact/ Mutilated and in pieces
Clothings	
Medical intervention (if any)	
Built	Well/ Moderate/ Poor/ Emaciated
Nourishment/ Physique	Lean/ Medium/ Obese
Scars/ Tattoos/ Bedsores (if present)	
Skin	Pallor/ Jaundiced/ Pink/ Cyanosis
Facial appearance	Pale/ Normal/ Livid/ Cyanosed
Eyes Cornea Pupils Conjunctivae	Closed/ Half open/ Open Clear/ Hazy/ Opaque Arcus senilis: Absent/ Developing/ Fully developed Constricted/ Dilated Regular/ Irregular Pale/ Normal/ Congested/ Jaundiced/ Hemorrhagic
Nostrils	
Ears	
Mouth	
Teeth	
Tongue	
Oral cavity	
Circum-oral regions Lips Inner aspects of lips Frenulum	 Pale/ Cyanosed Intact/ Torn
Orifice Urethral Anal Vaginal (in females)	
Condition of limbs	
Rigor mortis	Developing/ Fully developed/ Passing off Mild/ Strong
Postmortem staining	Fixed/ Not fixed Areas present__________________
Decomposition changes Skin Face/ abdomen/ scrotum Foul smell Maggots	 Color changes of putrefaction/ Marbling/ Skin slippage Bloated/ Not bloated Present/ Absent Present/ Absent
Any other findings	

.... Signature of doctor

B. External Injuries	
(Mention type, shape, length × breadth × depth of each injury and its relation to important body landmark. Indicate which injuries are fresh and which are old and their duration)	
C. Internal Examination	
Head Scalp Skull Brain	
Neck	
Chest Ribs/ sternum/ chest wall Pleural cavities Lungs Right Left Pericardium Heart Coronaries Large blood vessels	
Abdomen Peritoneum Stomach and its contents Small intestines its contents Large intestines and its contents Liver Gallbladder Spleen Pancreas Kidneys and ureters Urinary bladder Pelvic cavity	

* Injuries are to be given in serial number and mark them on the diagrams attached. In stab injuries, mention angles, margins and direction inside the body. In firearms injuries, mention direction and effects of fire.

……………………Signature of the doctor

Genital organs	
Spinal columns and spinal cord (opened where indicated)	

OPINION

a. Probable time since death (keeping all factors including observations at inquest)
   i. Between injury and death ____________________
   ii. Between death and postmortem examination ____________________
b. Cause and manner of death. The cause of death to the best of my knowledge and belief is:
   i. Immediate cause ____________________
   ii. Due to ____________________
   iii. Which of the injuries are antemortem/ postmortem and duration if antemortem? ____________________
   ____
   iv. Manner of causation of injuries (if possible) ____________________
   v. Whether injuries (individually or collectively) are sufficient to cause death in ordinary course of nature or not? ____________________
c. Any other ____________________

Specimens collected and preserved *(Tick '√')*

- ☐ Viscera (1. Stomach and small intestines with its contents, 2. Part of liver, half of each kidneys, spleen 3. Blood 4. Urine 5. Preservative used for sample 1 and 2, 6. Preservative used for sample 3 and 4)
- ☐ Sample of blood in gauze piece (dried)
- ☐ Clothes (air dried)
- ☐ Photographs/ Video CD in case of custody deaths/ Fingerprints
- ☐ Foreign body (like bullet, ligature)
- ☐ Slides from vagina or any other material ____________________
- ☐ Organs for histopathological examination

Place __________

____
Signature of the Doctor
Name (block letters), Designation and Seal

Received PM report No. ____________________ in original/copy along with body diagram and ____________________ inquest papers (mention total number and initial them all).

(Viscera or any other specimen, if preserved is handed over to the police immediately after autopsy)

Name ____________________ P.C. No. ____________________ P.S. ____________________

____
Signature and date

Date ______________ **PMR No.** ______________

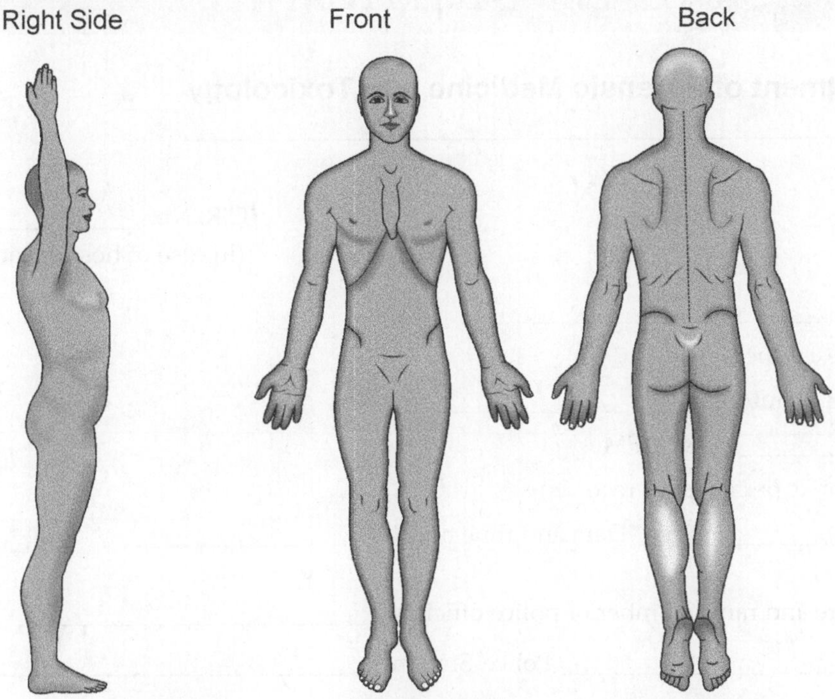

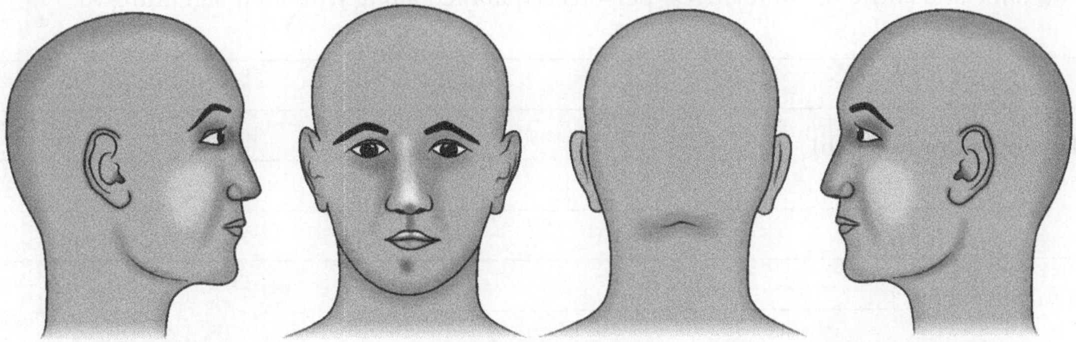

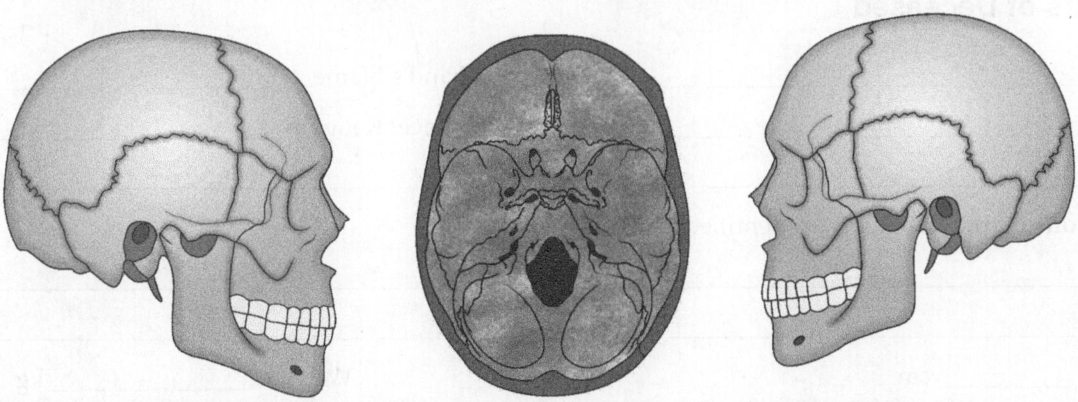

____
Signature of the Doctor
Name, Designation and Seal

EX. 7.5.6: POSTMORTEM REPORT

Department of Forensic Medicine and Toxicology

____

P.M. Report No. ____________ C.R. No. ____________
(in case of hospital admission)

Date and time of receipt of body ____________
Date and time of receipt of inquest papers ____________
Date and time of commencement of autopsy ____________
Time of completion of autopsy ________ AM/PM
In case of hospital deaths (particular as per hospital records)
Date and time of admission ____________ Date and time of death ____________

Body brought by (Name, signature and rank/ number of police official) ____________
____________ Police Station ____________

Identified by (Name and addresses of relatives/ persons acquainted along with their signature)

1. ____________
2. ____________

History (all events prior to death) ____________
____
____

Information furnished by: ____________

Particulars of Deceased

Name ____________ Father's/ Husband's Name ____________
Sex ____________ Age ____________ Race/ Religion ____________
Address ____________

Identifications marks (if body is unidentified)

1. ____________
2. ____________

Height ________ cm Weight ________ kg
Circumcision: Yes/ No Beard, mustache ____________

.... Signature of the doctor

SCHEDULE OF OBSERVATIONS

A. General	
Body	Entire and intact/ Mutilated and in pieces
Clothings	
Medical intervention (if any)	
Built	Well/ Moderate/ Poor/ Emaciated
Nourishment/ Physique	Lean/ Medium/ Obese
Scars/ Tattoos/ Bedsores (if present)	
Skin	Pallor/ Jaundiced/ Pink/ Cyanosis
Facial appearance	Pale/ Normal/ Livid/ Cyanosed
Eyes Cornea Pupils Conjunctivae	Closed/ Half open/ Open Clear/ Hazy/ Opaque Arcus senilis: Absent/ Developing/ Fully developed Constricted/ Dilated Regular/ Irregular Pale/ Normal/ Congested/ Jaundiced/ Hemorrhagic
Nostrils	
Ears	
Mouth	
Teeth	
Tongue	
Oral cavity	
Circum-oral regions Lips Inner aspects of lips Frenulum	 Pale/ Cyanosed Intact/ Torn
Orifice Urethral Anal Vaginal (in females)	
Condition of limbs	
Rigor mortis	Developing/ Fully developed/ Passing off Mild/ Strong
Postmortem staining	Fixed/ Not fixed Areas present____________________
Decomposition changes Skin Face/ abdomen/ scrotum Foul smell Maggots	 Color changes of putrefaction/ Marbling/ Skin slippage Bloated/ Not bloated Present/ Absent Present/ Absent
Any other findings	

.... Signature of doctor

B. External Injuries	
(Mention type, shape, length × breadth × depth of each injury and its relation to important body landmark. Indicate which injuries are fresh and which are old and their duration)	
C. Internal Examination	
Head Scalp Skull Brain	
Neck	
Chest Ribs/ sternum/ chest wall Pleural cavities Lungs Right Left Pericardium Heart Coronaries Large blood vessels	
Abdomen Peritoneum Stomach and its contents Small intestines its contents Large intestines and its contents Liver Gallbladder Spleen Pancreas Kidneys and ureters Urinary bladder Pelvic cavity	

* Injuries are to be given in serial number and mark them on the diagrams attached. In stab injuries, mention angles, margins and direction inside the body. In firearms injuries, mention direction and effects of fire.

......................Signature of the doctor

Genital organs	
Spinal columns and spinal cord (opened where indicated)	

OPINION

a. Probable time since death (keeping all factors including observations at inquest)

  i. Between injury and death ______

  ii. Between death and postmortem examination ______

b. Cause and manner of death. The cause of death to the best of my knowledge and belief is:

  i. Immediate cause ______

  ii. Due to ______

  iii. Which of the injuries are antemortem/ postmortem and duration if antemortem? ______

  ______

  iv. Manner of causation of injuries (if possible) ______

  v. Whether injuries (individually or collectively) are sufficient to cause death in ordinary course of nature or not? ______

c. Any other ______

Specimens collected and preserved *(Tick '√')*

- ☐ Viscera (1. Stomach and small intestines with its contents, 2. Part of liver, half of each kidneys, spleen 3. Blood 4. Urine 5. Preservative used for sample 1 and 2, 6. Preservative used for sample 3 and 4)
- ☐ Sample of blood in gauze piece (dried)
- ☐ Clothes (air dried)
- ☐ Photographs/ Video CD in case of custody deaths/ Fingerprints
- ☐ Foreign body (like bullet, ligature)
- ☐ Slides from vagina or any other material ______
- ☐ Organs for histopathological examination

______

Place ______

Signature of the Doctor
Name (block letters), Designation and Seal

Received PM report No. ______ in original/copy along with body diagram and ______ inquest papers (mention total number and initial them all).

(Viscera or any other specimen, if preserved is handed over to the police immediately after autopsy)

Name ______ P.C. No. ______ P.S. ______

______

Signature and date

Date ________________ PMR No. ________________

Right Side Front Back Left Side

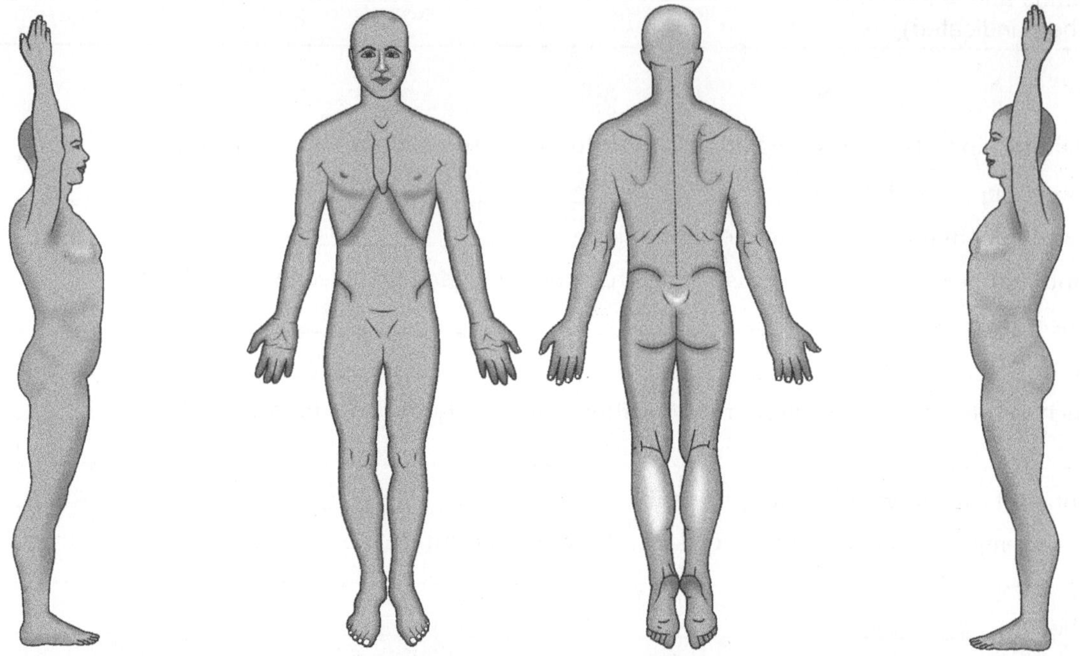

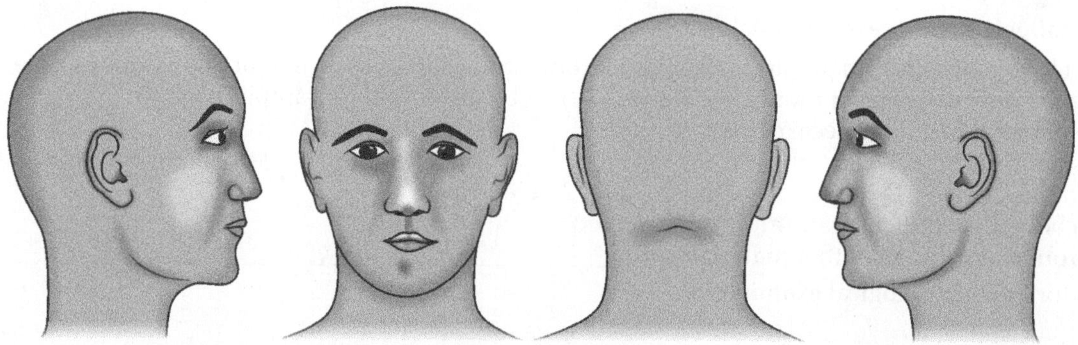

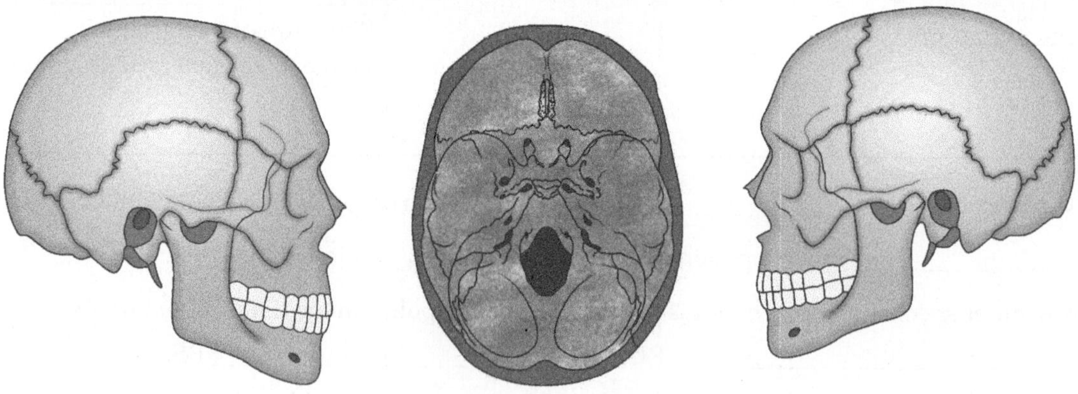

____

Signature of the Doctor
Name, Designation and Seal

EX. 7.5.7: POSTMORTEM REPORT

Department of Forensic Medicine and Toxicology

____

P.M. Report No. ______________ C.R. No. ______________ (in case of hospital admission)

Date and time of receipt of body ______________________

Date and time of receipt of inquest papers ______________

Date and time of commencement of autopsy ______________________

Time of completion of autopsy __________ AM/PM

In case of hospital deaths (particular as per hospital records)

Date and time of admission ______________ Date and time of death ______________

Body brought by (Name, signature and rank/ number of police official) ______________________

______________________________ Police Station ______________________

Identified by (Name and addresses of relatives/ persons acquainted along with their signature)

1. ____

2. ____

History (all events prior to death) ______________________________

____

____

Information furnished by: ______________________________

Particulars of Deceased

Name ______________________ Father's/ Husband's Name ______________________

Sex ______________ Age ______________ Race/ Religion ______________

Address ____

Identifications marks (if body is unidentified)

1. ____

2. ____

Height __________ cm Weight __________ kg

Circumcision: Yes/ No Beard, mustache ______________

.... Signature of the doctor

SCHEDULE OF OBSERVATIONS

A. General	
Body	Entire and intact/ Mutilated and in pieces
Clothings	
Medical intervention (if any)	
Built	Well/ Moderate/ Poor/ Emaciated
Nourishment/ Physique	Lean/ Medium/ Obese
Scars/ Tattoos/ Bedsores (if present)	
Skin	Pallor/ Jaundiced/ Pink/ Cyanosis
Facial appearance	Pale/ Normal/ Livid/ Cyanosed
Eyes Cornea Pupils Conjunctivae	Closed/ Half open/ Open Clear/ Hazy/ Opaque Arcus senilis: Absent/ Developing/ Fully developed Constricted/ Dilated Regular/ Irregular Pale/ Normal/ Congested/ Jaundiced/ Hemorrhagic
Nostrils	
Ears	
Mouth	
Teeth	
Tongue	
Oral cavity	
Circum-oral regions Lips Inner aspects of lips Frenulum	 Pale/ Cyanosed Intact/ Torn
Orifice Urethral Anal Vaginal (in females)	
Condition of limbs	
Rigor mortis	Developing/ Fully developed/ Passing off Mild/ Strong
Postmortem staining	Fixed/ Not fixed Areas present_______________
Decomposition changes Skin Face/ abdomen/ scrotum Foul smell Maggots	 Color changes of putrefaction/ Marbling/ Skin slippage Bloated/ Not bloated Present/ Absent Present/ Absent
Any other findings	

.... Signature of doctor

B. External Injuries
(Mention type, shape, length × breadth × depth of each injury and its relation to important body landmark. Indicate which injuries are fresh and which are old and their duration)

C. Internal Examination	
Head Scalp Skull Brain	
Neck	
Chest Ribs/ sternum/ chest wall Pleural cavities Lungs Right Left Pericardium Heart Coronaries Large blood vessels	
Abdomen Peritoneum Stomach and its contents Small intestines its contents Large intestines and its contents Liver Gallbladder Spleen Pancreas Kidneys and ureters Urinary bladder Pelvic cavity	

* Injuries are to be given in serial number and mark them on the diagrams attached. In stab injuries, mention angles, margins and direction inside the body. In firearms injuries, mention direction and effects of fire.

…………………..Signature of the doctor

Genital organs	
Spinal columns and spinal cord (opened where indicated)	

OPINION

a. Probable time since death (keeping all factors including observations at inquest)
   i. Between injury and death ____________________
   ii. Between death and postmortem examination ____________________

b. Cause and manner of death. The cause of death to the best of my knowledge and belief is:
   i. Immediate cause ____________________
   ii. Due to ____________________
   iii. Which of the injuries are antemortem/ postmortem and duration if antemortem? ____________________
   ____
   iv. Manner of causation of injuries (if possible) ____________________
   v. Whether injuries (individually or collectively) are sufficient to cause death in ordinary course of nature or not? ____________________

c. Any other ____________________

Specimens collected and preserved *(Tick '√')*

☐ Viscera (1. Stomach and small intestines with its contents, 2. Part of liver, half of each kidneys, spleen 3. Blood 4. Urine 5. Preservative used for sample 1 and 2, 6. Preservative used for sample 3 and 4)
☐ Sample of blood in gauze piece (dried)
☐ Clothes (air dried)
☐ Photographs/ Video CD in case of custody deaths/ Fingerprints
☐ Foreign body (like bullet, ligature)
☐ Slides from vagina or any other material ____________________
☐ Organs for histopathological examination

Place __________

____
Signature of the Doctor
Name (block letters), Designation and Seal

Received PM report No. ____________________ in original/copy along with body diagram and ____________________ inquest papers (mention total number and initial them all).

(Viscera or any other specimen, if preserved is handed over to the police immediately after autopsy)

Name ____________________ P.C. No. ____________________ P.S. ____________________

____
Signature and date

Date _______________ **PMR No.** _______________

Right Side Front Back Left Side

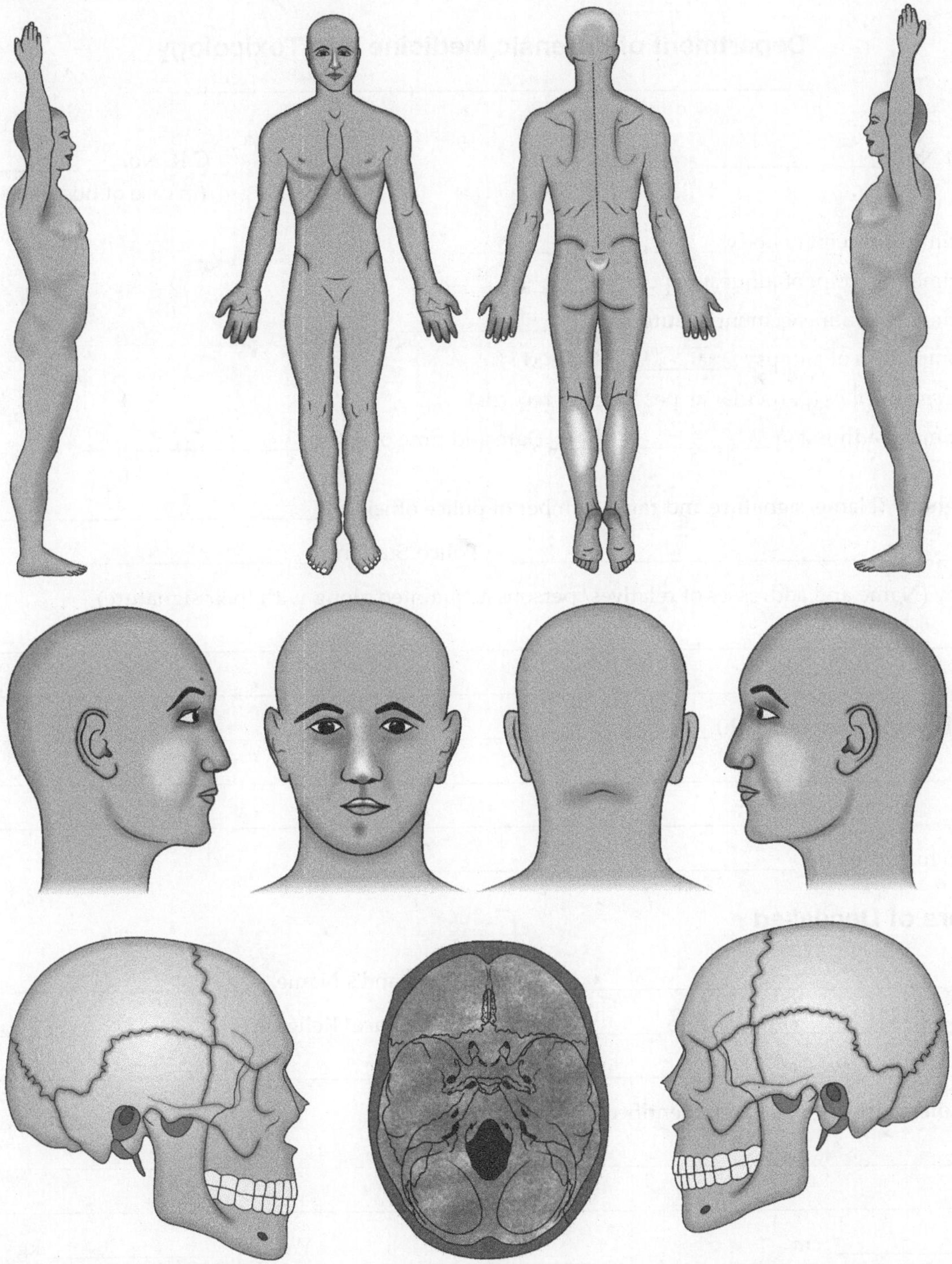

____

Signature of the Doctor
Name, Designation and Seal

EX. 7.5.8: POSTMORTEM REPORT

Department of Forensic Medicine and Toxicology

____

P.M. Report No. ______________

C.R. No. ______________
(in case of hospital admission)

Date and time of receipt of body ______________

Date and time of receipt of inquest papers ______________

Date and time of commencement of autopsy ______________

Time of completion of autopsy __________ AM/PM

In case of hospital deaths (particular as per hospital records)

Date and time of admission ______________ Date and time of death ______________

Body brought by (Name, signature and rank/ number of police official) ______________

______________ Police Station ______________

Identified by (Name and addresses of relatives/ persons acquainted along with their signature)

1. ______________
2. ______________

History (all events prior to death) ______________

____

____

Information furnished by: ______________

Particulars of Deceased

Name ______________ Father's/ Husband's Name ______________

Sex ______________ Age ______________ Race/ Religion ______________

Address ______________

Identifications marks (if body is unidentified)

1. ______________
2. ______________

Height ______________ cm

Weight ______________ kg

Circumcision: Yes/ No

Beard, mustache ______________

.... Signature of the doctor

SCHEDULE OF OBSERVATIONS

A. General	
Body	Entire and intact/ Mutilated and in pieces
Clothings	
Medical intervention (if any)	
Built	Well/ Moderate/ Poor/ Emaciated
Nourishment/ Physique	Lean/ Medium/ Obese
Scars/ Tattoos/ Bedsores (if present)	
Skin	Pallor/ Jaundiced/ Pink/ Cyanosis
Facial appearance	Pale/ Normal/ Livid/ Cyanosed
Eyes Cornea Pupils Conjunctivae	Closed/ Half open/ Open Clear/ Hazy/ Opaque Arcus senilis: Absent/ Developing/ Fully developed Constricted/ Dilated Regular/ Irregular Pale/ Normal/ Congested/ Jaundiced/ Hemorrhagic
Nostrils	
Ears	
Mouth	
Teeth	
Tongue	
Oral cavity	
Circum-oral regions Lips Inner aspects of lips Frenulum	 Pale/ Cyanosed Intact/ Torn
Orifice Urethral Anal Vaginal (in females)	
Condition of limbs	
Rigor mortis	Developing/ Fully developed/ Passing off Mild/ Strong
Postmortem staining	Fixed/ Not fixed Areas present____________________
Decomposition changes Skin Face/ abdomen/ scrotum Foul smell Maggots	 Color changes of putrefaction/ Marbling/ Skin slippage Bloated/ Not bloated Present/ Absent Present/ Absent
Any other findings	

.... Signature of doctor

B. External Injuries
(Mention type, shape, length × breadth × depth of each injury and its relation to important body landmark. Indicate which injuries are fresh and which are old and their duration)

C. Internal Examination	
Head Scalp Skull Brain	
Neck	
Chest Ribs/ sternum/ chest wall Pleural cavities Lungs Right Left Pericardium Heart Coronaries Large blood vessels	
Abdomen Peritoneum Stomach and its contents Small intestines its contents Large intestines and its contents Liver Gallbladder Spleen Pancreas Kidneys and ureters Urinary bladder Pelvic cavity	

* Injuries are to be given in serial number and mark them on the diagrams attached. In stab injuries, mention angles, margins and direction inside the body. In firearms injuries, mention direction and effects of fire.

……………………Signature of the doctor

Genital organs	
Spinal columns and spinal cord (opened where indicated)	

OPINION

a. Probable time since death (keeping all factors including observations at inquest)

   i. Between injury and death ____________________

   ii. Between death and postmortem examination ____________________

b. Cause and manner of death. The cause of death to the best of my knowledge and belief is:

   i. Immediate cause ____________________

   ii. Due to ____________________

   iii. Which of the injuries are antemortem/ postmortem and duration if antemortem? ____________________

   ____

   iv. Manner of causation of injuries (if possible) ____________________

   v. Whether injuries (individually or collectively) are sufficient to cause death in ordinary course of nature or not? ____________________

c. Any other ____________________

Specimens collected and preserved *(Tick '√')*

- ☐ Viscera (1. Stomach and small intestines with its contents, 2. Part of liver, half of each kidneys, spleen 3. Blood 4. Urine 5. Preservative used for sample 1 and 2, 6. Preservative used for sample 3 and 4)
- ☐ Sample of blood in gauze piece (dried)
- ☐ Clothes (air dried)
- ☐ Photographs/ Video CD in case of custody deaths/ Fingerprints
- ☐ Foreign body (like bullet, ligature)
- ☐ Slides from vagina or any other material ____________________
- ☐ Organs for histopathological examination

Place __________

____

Signature of the Doctor

Name (block letters), Designation and Seal

Received PM report No. ____________________ in original/copy along with body diagram and ____________________ inquest papers (mention total number and initial them all).

(Viscera or any other specimen, if preserved is handed over to the police immediately after autopsy)

Name ____________________ P.C. No. ____________________ P.S. ____________________

____

Signature and date

Date ______________ PMR No. ____________

Right Side Front Back Left Side

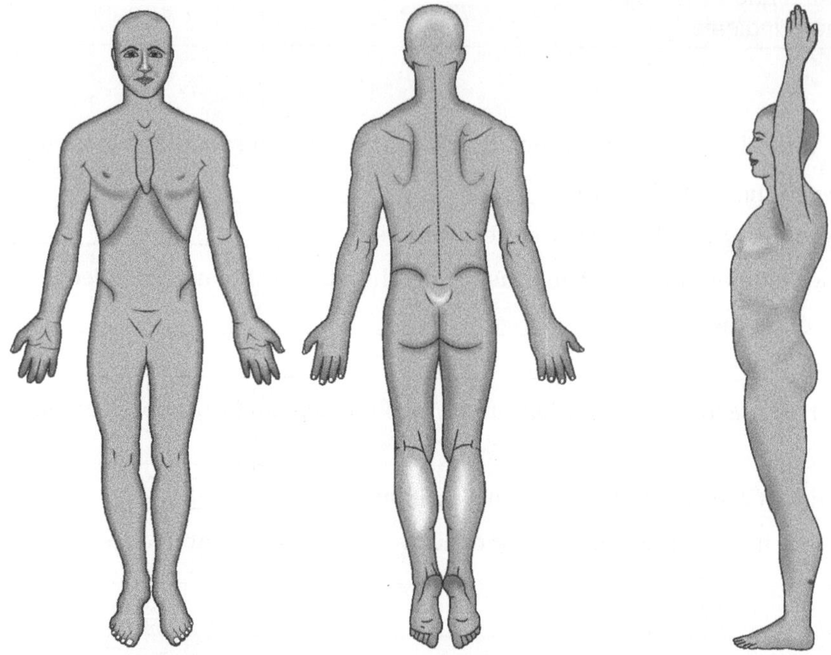

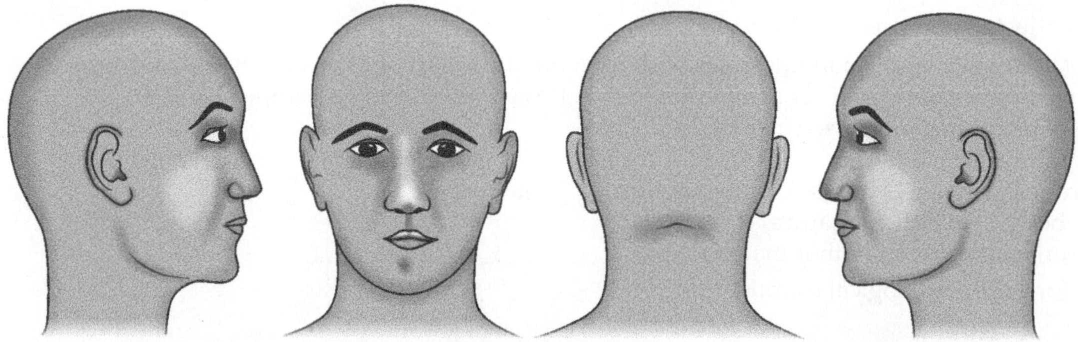

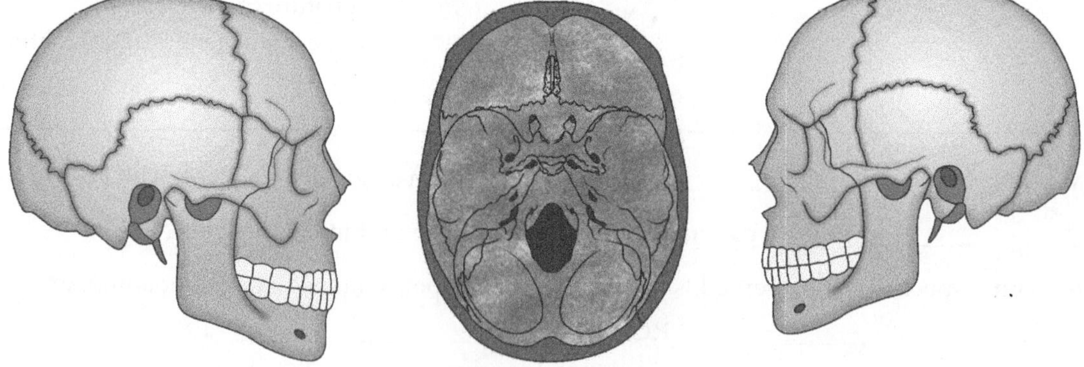

____

Signature of the Doctor
Name, Designation and Seal

EX. 7.5.9: POSTMORTEM REPORT

Department of Forensic Medicine and Toxicology

____

P.M. Report No. ________________ C.R. No. ________________ (in case of hospital admission)

Date and time of receipt of body ______________________

Date and time of receipt of inquest papers ________________

Date and time of commencement of autopsy ____________________

Time of completion of autopsy __________ AM/PM

In case of hospital deaths (particular as per hospital records)

Date and time of admission ________________ Date and time of death ________________

Body brought by (Name, signature and rank/ number of police official) ______________________________

____ Police Station ________________________________

Identified by (Name and addresses of relatives/ persons acquainted along with their signature)

1. ____
2. ____

History (all events prior to death) ____

____

____

Information furnished by: ____________________________________

Particulars of Deceased

Name ______________________________________ Father's/ Husband's Name ________________________________

Sex __________________________ Age ______________________ Race/ Religion ____________________________

Address ____

Identifications marks (if body is unidentified)

1. ____
2. ____

Height ____________ cm Weight ________________ kg

Circumcision: Yes/ No Beard, mustache ____________________

.... Signature of the doctor

SCHEDULE OF OBSERVATIONS

A. General	
Body	Entire and intact/ Mutilated and in pieces
Clothings	
Medical intervention (if any)	
Built	Well/ Moderate/ Poor/ Emaciated
Nourishment/ Physique	Lean/ Medium/ Obese
Scars/ Tattoos/ Bedsores (if present)	
Skin	Pallor/ Jaundiced/ Pink/ Cyanosis
Facial appearance	Pale/ Normal/ Livid/ Cyanosed
Eyes Cornea Pupils Conjunctivae	Closed/ Half open/ Open Clear/ Hazy/ Opaque Arcus senilis: Absent/ Developing/ Fully developed Constricted/ Dilated Regular/ Irregular Pale/ Normal/ Congested/ Jaundiced/ Hemorrhagic
Nostrils	
Ears	
Mouth	
Teeth	
Tongue	
Oral cavity	
Circum-oral regions Lips Inner aspects of lips Frenulum	 Pale/ Cyanosed Intact/ Torn
Orifice Urethral Anal Vaginal (in females)	
Condition of limbs	
Rigor mortis	Developing/ Fully developed/ Passing off Mild/ Strong
Postmortem staining	Fixed/ Not fixed Areas present__________________
Decomposition changes Skin Face/ abdomen/ scrotum Foul smell Maggots	 Color changes of putrefaction/ Marbling/ Skin slippage Bloated/ Not bloated Present/ Absent Present/ Absent
Any other findings	

.... Signature of doctor

B. External Injuries
(Mention type, shape, length × breadth × depth of each injury and its relation to important body landmark. Indicate which injuries are fresh and which are old and their duration)

C. Internal Examination	
Head Scalp Skull Brain	
Neck	
Chest Ribs/ sternum/ chest wall Pleural cavities Lungs Right Left Pericardium Heart Coronaries Large blood vessels	
Abdomen Peritoneum Stomach and its contents Small intestines its contents Large intestines and its contents Liver Gallbladder Spleen Pancreas Kidneys and ureters Urinary bladder Pelvic cavity	

* Injuries are to be given in serial number and mark them on the diagrams attached. In stab injuries, mention angles, margins and direction inside the body. In firearms injuries, mention direction and effects of fire.

…………………Signature of the doctor

Genital organs	
Spinal columns and spinal cord (opened where indicated)	

OPINION

a. Probable time since death (keeping all factors including observations at inquest)
   i. Between injury and death ____________
   ii. Between death and postmortem examination ____________

b. Cause and manner of death. The cause of death to the best of my knowledge and belief is:
   i. Immediate cause ____________
   ii. Due to ____________
   iii. Which of the injuries are antemortem/ postmortem and duration if antemortem? ____________
   ____
   iv. Manner of causation of injuries (if possible) ____________
   v. Whether injuries (individually or collectively) are sufficient to cause death in ordinary course of nature or not? ____________

c. Any other ____________

Specimens collected and preserved *(Tick '√')*

☐ Viscera (1. Stomach and small intestines with its contents, 2. Part of liver, half of each kidneys, spleen 3. Blood 4. Urine 5. Preservative used for sample 1 and 2, 6. Preservative used for sample 3 and 4)
☐ Sample of blood in gauze piece (dried)
☐ Clothes (air dried)
☐ Photographs/ Video CD in case of custody deaths/ Fingerprints
☐ Foreign body (like bullet, ligature)
☐ Slides from vagina or any other material ____________
☐ Organs for histopathological examination

Place ________

____
Signature of the Doctor
Name (block letters), Designation and Seal

Received PM report No. ____________ in original/copy along with body diagram and ____________ inquest papers (mention total number and initial them all).

(Viscera or any other specimen, if preserved is handed over to the police immediately after autopsy)

Name ____________ P.C. No. ____________ P.S. ____________

____
Signature and date

Date ______________ **PMR No.** ______________

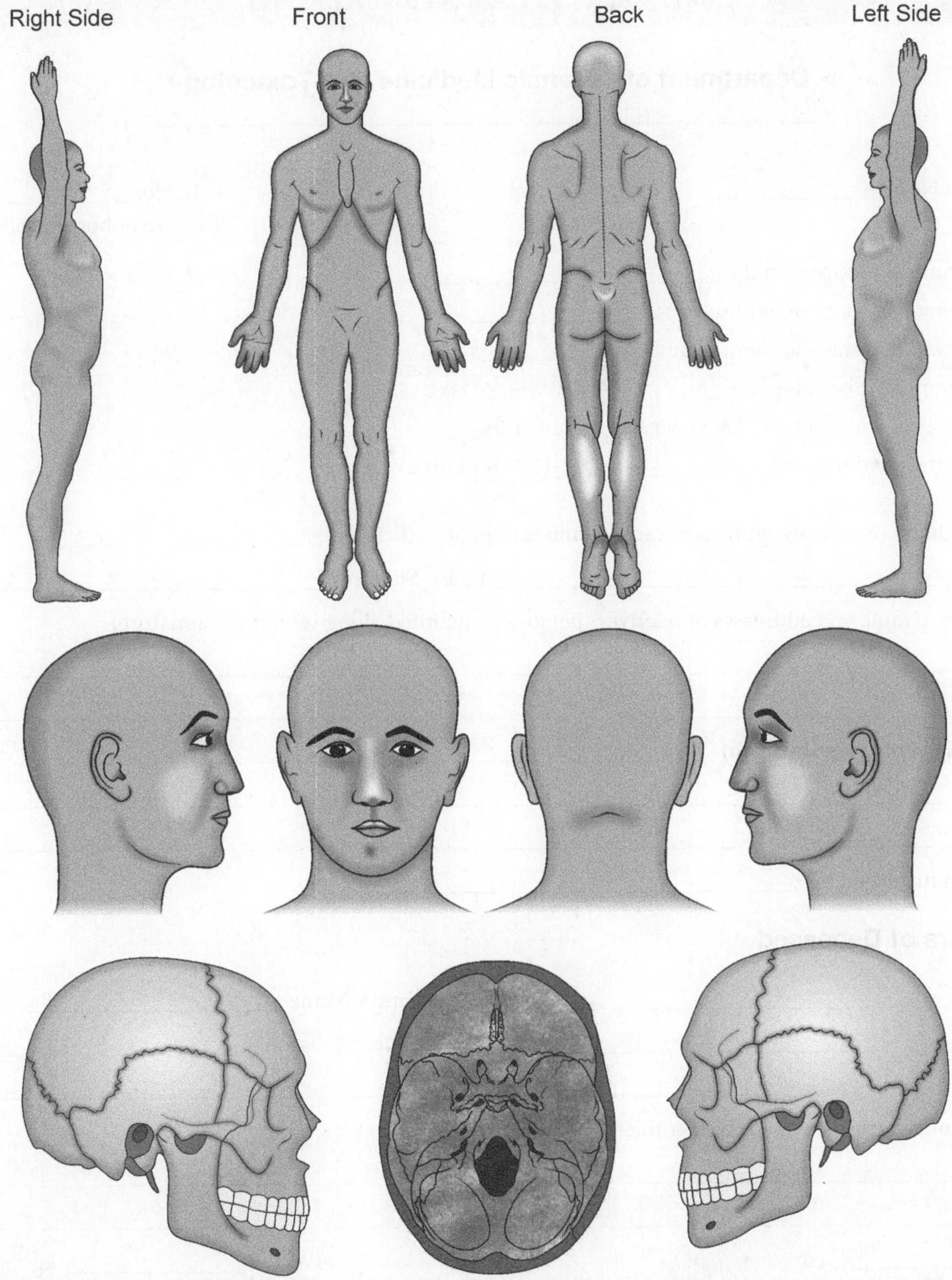

____

Signature of the Doctor
Name, Designation and Seal

EX. 7.5.10: POSTMORTEM REPORT

Department of Forensic Medicine and Toxicology

____

P.M. Report No. ________________ C.R. No. ________________
(in case of hospital admission)

Date and time of receipt of body ______________________
Date and time of receipt of inquest papers ________________
Date and time of commencement of autopsy ______________________
Time of completion of autopsy __________ AM/PM
In case of hospital deaths (particular as per hospital records)
Date and time of admission ________________ Date and time of death ________________

Body brought by (Name, signature and rank/ number of police official) ______________________
______________________________ Police Station ______________________
Identified by (Name and addresses of relatives/ persons acquainted along with their signature)
1. ______________________________
2. ______________________________

History (all events prior to death) ______________________________
____
____

Information furnished by: ______________________

Particulars of Deceased

Name ______________________ Father's/ Husband's Name ______________________
Sex ________________ Age ________________ Race/ Religion ________________
Address ______________________________

Identifications marks (if body is unidentified)
1. ______________________________
2. ______________________________

Height ____________ cm Weight ____________ kg
Circumcision: Yes/ No Beard, mustache ____________

.... Signature of the doctor

SCHEDULE OF OBSERVATIONS

A. General	
Body	Entire and intact/ Mutilated and in pieces
Clothings	
Medical intervention (if any)	
Built	Well/ Moderate/ Poor/ Emaciated
Nourishment/ Physique	Lean/ Medium/ Obese
Scars/ Tattoos/ Bedsores (if present)	
Skin	Pallor/ Jaundiced/ Pink/ Cyanosis
Facial appearance	Pale/ Normal/ Livid/ Cyanosed
Eyes Cornea Pupils Conjunctivae	Closed/ Half open/ Open Clear/ Hazy/ Opaque Arcus senilis: Absent/ Developing/ Fully developed Constricted/ Dilated Regular/ Irregular Pale/ Normal/ Congested/ Jaundiced/ Hemorrhagic
Nostrils	
Ears	
Mouth	
Teeth	
Tongue	
Oral cavity	
Circum-oral regions Lips Inner aspects of lips Frenulum	 Pale/ Cyanosed Intact/ Torn
Orifice Urethral Anal Vaginal (in females)	
Condition of limbs	
Rigor mortis	Developing/ Fully developed/ Passing off Mild/ Strong
Postmortem staining	Fixed/ Not fixed Areas present__________________
Decomposition changes Skin Face/ abdomen/ scrotum Foul smell Maggots	 Color changes of putrefaction/ Marbling/ Skin slippage Bloated/ Not bloated Present/ Absent Present/ Absent
Any other findings	

.... Signature of doctor

B. External Injuries
(Mention type, shape, length × breadth × depth of each injury and its relation to important body landmark. Indicate which injuries are fresh and which are old and their duration)

C. Internal Examination	
Head Scalp Skull Brain	
Neck	
Chest Ribs/ sternum/ chest wall Pleural cavities Lungs Right Left Pericardium Heart Coronaries Large blood vessels	
Abdomen Peritoneum Stomach and its contents Small intestines its contents Large intestines and its contents Liver Gallbladder Spleen Pancreas Kidneys and ureters Urinary bladder Pelvic cavity	

* Injuries are to be given in serial number and mark them on the diagrams attached. In stab injuries, mention angles, margins and direction inside the body. In firearms injuries, mention direction and effects of fire.

……………………Signature of the doctor

Genital organs	
Spinal columns and spinal cord (opened where indicated)	

OPINION

a. Probable time since death (keeping all factors including observations at inquest)

   i. Between injury and death ______

   ii. Between death and postmortem examination ______

b. Cause and manner of death. The cause of death to the best of my knowledge and belief is:

   i. Immediate cause ______

   ii. Due to ______

   iii. Which of the injuries are antemortem/ postmortem and duration if antemortem? ______

   ______

   iv. Manner of causation of injuries (if possible) ______

   v. Whether injuries (individually or collectively) are sufficient to cause death in ordinary course of nature or not? ______

c. Any other ______

Specimens collected and preserved *(Tick '√')*

- ☐ Viscera (1. Stomach and small intestines with its contents, 2. Part of liver, half of each kidneys, spleen 3. Blood 4. Urine 5. Preservative used for sample 1 and 2, 6. Preservative used for sample 3 and 4)
- ☐ Sample of blood in gauze piece (dried)
- ☐ Clothes (air dried)
- ☐ Photographs/ Video CD in case of custody deaths/ Fingerprints
- ☐ Foreign body (like bullet, ligature)
- ☐ Slides from vagina or any other material ______
- ☐ Organs for histopathological examination

______

Place ______

Signature of the Doctor
Name (block letters), Designation and Seal

Received PM report No. ______ in original/copy along with body diagram and ______ inquest papers (mention total number and initial them all).

(Viscera or any other specimen, if preserved is handed over to the police immediately after autopsy)

Name ______ P.C. No. ______ P.S. ______

______

Signature and date

Date ____________ PMR No. ____________

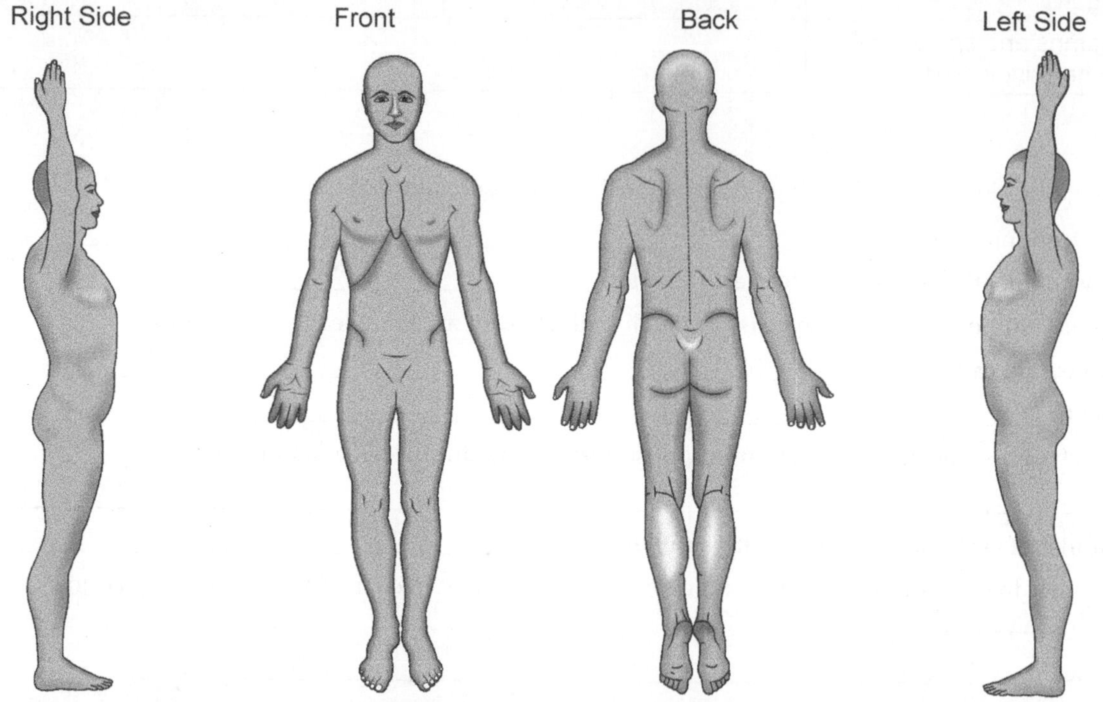

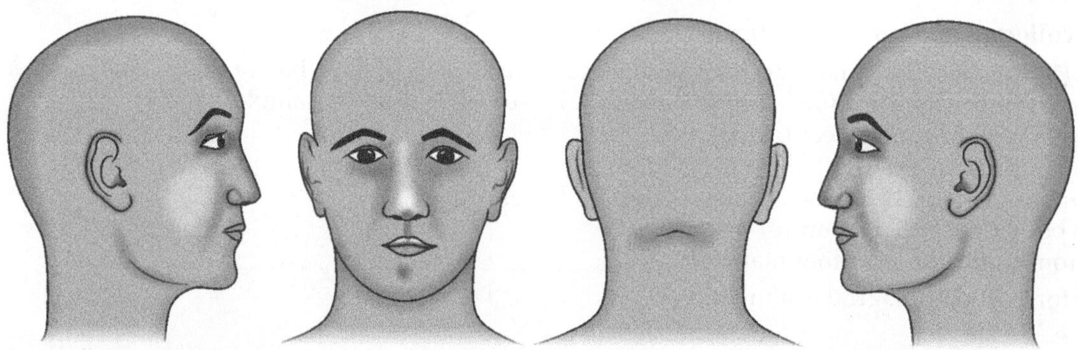

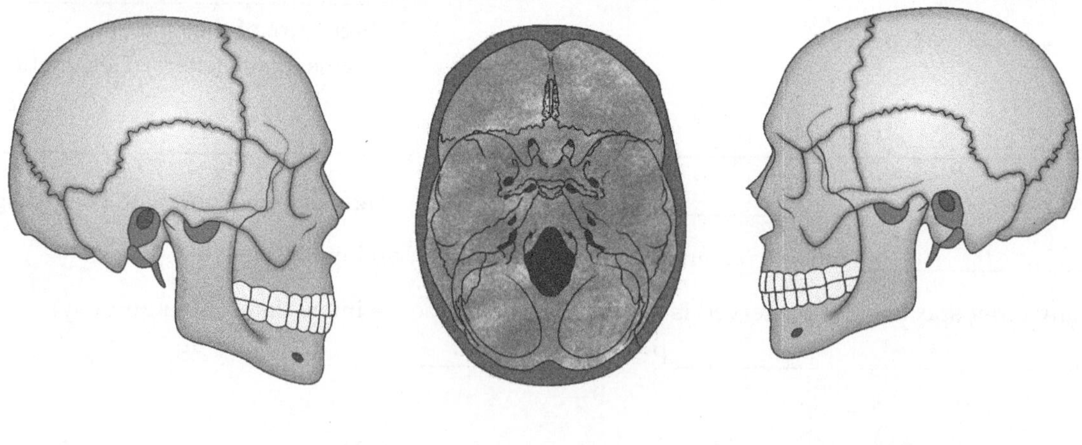

Signature of the Doctor
Name, Designation and Seal

LABELS TO BE ATTACHED TO MATERIAL SENT FOR CHEMICAL ANALYSIS

Department of Forensic Medicine and Toxicology

____

Viscera/ Blood for Chemical Analysis

P.M. No.______________ Date ______________

Bottle No. ____________

Name of the deceased __________________________________ Age __________ years Sex: ____________

Contents of this bottle: ____

Preservative: Saturated solution of sodium chloride/ Sodium fluoride

Signature of the Medical Officer

Department of Forensic Medicine and Toxicology

____

Sample preservative

P.M. No.______________ Date ______________

Bottle No. ____________

Name of the deceased __________________________________ Age __________ years Sex: ____________

Contents of this bottle: Saturated solution of sodium chloride/ Sodium fluoride (preservative used)

Signature of the Medical Officer

LABEL TO BE AFFIXED ON THE SEALED BOX OF VISCERA

Department of Forensic Medicine and Toxicology

____

Materials: 1. Stomach, intestine and its contents, 2. Part of liver and half of each kidney, 3. Blood, 4. Urine, 5. Saturated solution of saline, 5. Sodium fluoride

P.M. No ______________ Date: ____________

Name of the deceased: __________________ Age ________________ years Sex: ___________________

FIR No. ______________________ of ____ police station.

Place: _____________

____

Signature of the Medical Officer
Name, Designation and Seal

EX. 7.6: REPORT FORWARDED WITH THE VISCERA SENT FOR CHEMICAL ANALYSIS

Department of Forensic Medicine and Toxicology

____

To

The Chemical Examiner

Govt. of ______________

______________ (District/City)

Subject: Viscera for chemical analysis for suspected ______________ poisoning

Sir/ Madam

I am forwarding the case particulars and below mentioned material through

Mr. ______________ P.C. No ______________ for chemical analysis and certificate.

P.M. No. ______________ Dated: ______________

Name of the deceased: ______________ Age ________ years, Sex ________

FIR No. ______________ of ______________ police station.

Materials:

a. A cloth covered sealed box with 10 seals containing:
   1. Stomach and part of intestine with its contents
   2. Part of liver and one half of each kidney
   3. Blood
   4. Urine
   5. Saturated saline (sample of preservative for 1 and 2)
   6. Sodium fluoride (sample of preservative for 3 and 4)

b. A sealed envelope with 5 seals containing
   1. Request for chemical analysis
   2. Copy of PM report
   3. ________ number of inquest papers duly signed
   4. Sample seal

Alleged cause of death as per inquest ______________

Poisoning/ drug suspected ______________

Examination required: Quantitative and qualitative analysis for drugs/ poisons suspected.

I request you that the report may be sent to the undersigned at the earliest.

Yours faithfully,

Signature of the Doctor

Name, Designation and Seal

Place ____________

Date ____________

EX. 7.7: REQUISITION FOR HISTOPATHOLOGICAL EXAMINATION

Department of Forensic Medicine and Toxicology

____

To
The Professor/ Medical Officer I/ C
Department of Pathology
____

Subject: Histopathological examination of specimens preserved during the postmortem examination (Ref.: PM. No. ________ dated __________)

Sir/ Madam,

I request that the histopathological examination of the following specimens, preserved from the dead body of Mr/ Ms ______________________________, S/ D/ W of ______________________ aged __________ years, involved in FIR No __________ of __________ police station may be conducted, as the findings of such examination are absolutely necessary for furnishing opinion as to cause of death.

The alleged cause of death as per requisition for postmortem examination was ______________________________
____

Relevant findings at autopsy:

Organs/ Specimens sent: *(Tick '√')*

- ☐ Heart (whole, cut open)
- ☐ Brain (______________________)
- ☐ Lungs (______________________)
- ☐ Liver (______________________)
- ☐ Spleen (______________________)
- ☐ Kidneys (______________________)
- ☐ Pancreas (______________________)
- ☐ Female genitals (uterus, fallopian tubes, ovaries, vagina)
- ☐ Others (______________________________)

I am sending the specimens in sealed packet and preserved in 10% formalin through H.C./P.C. No. __________. I request you that the results of histopathology report may be made ready at the earliest, so as to be collected through police.

With regards,

____
Signature of the Doctor
Name, Designation and Seal

Place __________

Date __________

EX. 7.8: FINAL OPINION AS TO CAUSE OF DEATH

Department of Forensic Medicine and Toxicology

____

To

Date ____________

The Investigating Officer,

____________________Police Station

____________________ (District/ City)

Subject: Final opinion regarding PM report No. ______________ dated ______________

Ref:

a. Chemical Examiner's report no. ____________________________ dated ____________

b. Histopathology report no. ________________________ dated ____________

c. Microbiology/ Biochemistry report no. ____________________ dated ________

As per requisition from the ________________________________ of ________________

police station dated ________________________, postmortem examination was conducted on the body of Mr/ Ms __________________________________ S/ D/ W of ______________________________

aged about __________________ years, involved in FIR No. ____________ of ________________ police station and the P.M. report number ______________ dated ________ was issued by the undersigned.

The opinion as to cause of death was reserved pending results of chemical analysis of viscera and/ or other material objects preserved from the body. *(Strike off if not applicable)*

The certificate of chemical analysis number ______________dated ________of the above said viscera and other materials were received by me on ______________.

Opinion

Based on the postmortem findings and results of laboratory examinations, I am of the opinion that the cause of death in above mentioned case was:

i. Immediate cause ____

ii. Due to ____

____

Signature of the Doctor
Name, Designation and Seal

Place ________

Date ________

Received final opinion of PM report No. ______________.

Name________________________________ P.C.No.____________________ P.S.______________

____

Signature and date

NOTES

NOTES

UNIT VIII

Project
(Optional)

Case reports help students gain a deeper understanding of a topic—it serves as source of knowledge and important means for education and learning as he/ she has to search and read extensively on that topic. They also act as an excellent introduction to academic writing. Doing a literature review, structuring a manuscript and learning how to revise the article are skills worth developing during their undergraduate days. The students will find abstract medical knowledge easier to remember when linked to a subject/ patient. Case reports are generally related to unusual or previously unreported condition or findings. However, to keep it simple for the first time authors, this can be any case of that he/ she has seen during the emergency or autopsy posting.

The student is required to workup and submit one case report within the stipulated dead line announced by the department. This case report may include any road traffic accident, burns, electrocution, firearm injury, sharp force injury, blunt force injury, fall from height, sexual offences, impotency, poisoning or any other medicolegal case that he/ she has observed in the emergency. The autopsy case may include any accidental deaths, burns, hanging, strangulation, throttling, drowning, firearm deaths, sexual murder, fall from height, poisoning deaths, etc.

SCHEME OF WRITING THE REPORT

Important Considerations

1. *'De-identification' of the individual:* In order to maintain confidentiality, the patient's name, address and other identifiers such as hospital registration number must not be used. In photographs, masking (covering a subject's face or eyes) is done, and radiological images are anonymised to prevent identification.
2. *Obtain informed consent:* It is important to obtain written consent from the patient, if the student is taking any medicolegal case in the emergency. During the consent process, the student must explain the purpose of the study, and also take specific consent if he/ she wish to include photographs.
3. *Data collection:* Before beginning to write the case itself, the student should gather all of the materials relevant to the case—clinical notes, laboratory reports, X-rays, photographs, etc.–and form a clear picture of the case that he/ she wish to write. Once written, check the spelling and grammar.
4. *Literature review:* A literature review on a medical database such as PubMed, Med-Ind, Embase, Google Scholar or Medline can be used to check if there have been any similar cases. Previously published case reports will help improve understanding of the topic.

How to Write the Case Report

Case reports should encompass the following sections: title, abstract with keywords, introduction with a literature review, description of the case including a MLR or PMR, discussion that includes a detailed literature review and a conclusion. (Check list is given in Table 8.1)

Title

The first page of the project should be a dedicated to title page. The 'title' should be a clear and short description of the case along with student's full name, batch, roll no., institutional address and e-mail address. Abbreviations within the title should be avoided.

Abstract

It is better to write the abstract, once the main body of text has been completed. Abstracts should be concise, about 150–250 words. It summaries the case and gives an overall idea about the content of the case report. Abbreviations or references within the abstract should not be used.

Students can write the abstracts using one of two styles, *unstructured* (narrative) or *structured*. A narrative abstract consists of a short version of the whole paper. There are no headings within the narrative abstract. A structured abstract uses subheadings, and can be divided into three sections: Background: an introduction about this case; Case presentation: brief details of the case (brief history and findings); and Conclusions: brief conclusion of what the reader should learn from the case report.

Keywords

Provide 2–5 keywords which will be used when searching for the case report using a search engine.

Introduction

Briefly summarize the background and context of this case report. This should be from the standpoint of those without specialist knowledge in the area, explaining the background of the topic. If similar cases have been reported previously, describe them briefly. A more detailed literature review is done in the discussion. Each time, when referred to a previous study, cite the reference (usually at the end of the sentence, in superscripts).

Case Description

Write in a narrative style, restricting to the relevant information. The case report is best presented in chronological order, typically comprising of patient's demographic information (without any details that could lead to the identification of the patient), history of the incident, any relevant medical or past history of the patient, examination findings, starting with the vital signs presented at the examination, investigative results, including imaging and laboratory results, brief management and diagnosis.

All important negative findings should also be provided. Include two or three photographs to keep the reader engaged. Photographs should be of good quality along with scale and date. In the case of surgery and pathology consults, a comprehensive summary of the surgical procedure and detailed pathologist's report should be included. X-rays or other images are included, if they are clear enough to be easily reproduced.

- *Management and outcome:* Briefly describe the plan for care, as well as the care which was actually provided and the outcome.
- The medicolegal report or the postmortem report in proper format should be included in the report.
- Final opinion in medicolegal reports should be based on the diagnostic results (testing, imaging) and specialists' opinions (pathological reports, surgical reports, etc.) which should be given at the end of case description.

Discussion

The discussion is the most important section of the case report. It evaluates the case and compare and contrast with the published literature. Start by briefly expanding on introduction, then sum up the current literature related to the case. Describe what has already been reported about this topic, what are the main findings, explain those findings and how the present case differs or conforms to those previously published literature.

Give information about the condition in question, such as the definitions, basic epidemiology, pathophysiology, clinical presentation and investigations.

Further Research/ Suggestions

The student may give his/ her suggestions for further research. Lessons learnt from the case with justifiable evidence-based recommendations may be included.

Conclusions

State clearly the main conclusions of the case report and give a clear explanation of its importance and relevance.

Acknowldgments

Students should acknowledge anyone who contributed towards the article by making substantial contributions or who was involved in drafting the manuscript.

References

Students must search for and cite published case reports that are relevant to the case. References should be listed in the Vancouver or Harvard style. There should be not more than 15–20 current references (within the last 5 years, unless it is of historic interest). The Vancouver system of referencing is cited below:

Books

1. Author Surname Initials. Title: subtitle. Edition (if not the first). Place of publication: Publisher; Year.
    a. Mason J. Concepts in dental public health. Philadelphia: Lippincott Williams and Wilkins; 2005.
    b. Dionne RA, Phero JC, Becker DE (eds). Management of pain and anxiety in the dental office. Philadelphia: WB Saunders; 2002.
    c. Fauci AS, Braunwald E, Kasper DL, Hauser SL, Longo DL, Jameson JL, et al. (eds). Harrison's principles of internal medicine. 17th ed. New York: McGraw Hill; 2008. (if more than 6 authors/editors)

Chapter in a book

Alexander RG. Considerations in creating a beautiful smile. In: Romano R (ed). The art of the smile. London: Quintessence Publishing; 2005. p. 187-210.

E-book

Irfan A. Protocols for predictable aesthetic dental restorations [Internet]. Oxford: Blackwell Munksgaard; 2006 [cited 2009 May 21]. Available from Netlibrary: http://cclsw2.vcc.ca:2048/login?url=http://www.netLibrary.com/urlapi.asp?action=summary&v=1&bookid=181691

Organization as Author

Canadian Dental Hygienists Association. Dental hygiene: definition and scope. Ottawa: Canadian Dental Hygienists Association; 1995.

No Author/ Editor

Scott's Canadian dental directory 2008. 9th ed. Toronto: Scott's Directories; 2007.

Government Document

Canada. Environmental Health Directorate. Radiation protection in dentistry: recommended safety procedures for the use of dental X-ray equipment. Safety Code 30. Ottawa: Ministry of Health; 2000.

Format for Journal Articles

Author Surname Initials. Title of article. Title of journal, abbreviated. Date of Publication: Volume Number (Issue Number): Page Numbers.

Haas AN, de Castro GD, Moreno T, Susin C, Albandar JM, Oppermann RV, et al. Azithromycin as a adjunctive treatment of aggressive periodontitis: 12-months randomized clinical trial. J Clin Periodontol. 2008; 35(8): 696-704.

Journal Article from a Website

Tasdemir T, Yesilyurt C, Ceyhanli KT, Celik D, Er K. Evaluation of apical filling after root canal filling by 2 different techniques. J Can Dent Assoc [Internet]. 2009 [cited 2009 Jun 14];75(3):[about 5pp.]. Available from: http://www.cda-adc.ca/jcda/vol-75/issue-3/201.html

Dictionary, Encyclopedia or Similar Reference Book

Unsigned

Mosby's dental dictionary. 2nd ed. St. Louis: Mosby Elsevier; 2008. Frenotomy; p. 273.

Signed (and Online)

Murchison DF. Dental emergencies. In: Merck Manual of Diagnosis and Therapy [Internet]. 18th ed. Whitehouse Station (NJ): Merck; 2009 [last modified 2009 Mar; cited 2009 Jun 23]. Available from: http://www.merck.com/mmpe/sec08/ch096/ch096a.html?qt=dental&alt=sh

Newspaper Articles

1. Fayerman P. Women must now wait to 40 for publicly paid amnio test. Vancouver Sun. 2009 Jun 9; Sect. A: 5.
2. Health Canada issues warning over fake toothbrushes. The Globe and Mail [Internet]. 2009 April 10 [cited 2009 Jun 23]. Available from: http://www.theglobeandmail.com/news/national/health-canada-issues-warning-over-fake-toothbrushes/article973190/

Table 8.1: Checklist for writing case reports

Title
• Should be brief and informative.
Abstract
• Word limit of 150–250 words.
• No abbreviations, no references.
Introduction
• Should be concise and attract the reader's attention.
• Similar cases that have been reported previously are described briefly.
Case report
• Describe the history of the incident.
• Provide details of the presentation and examination, including those from imaging and laboratory studies. Describe briefly the treatment and diagnosis.
• Provide details of the examination findings in postmortem report.
• Fill up the medicolegal report or postmortem report in proper format.
• Figures, illustrations, photographs, tables, X-rays, CT scans, etc.
• Informed consent form (in medicolegal reports).
Discussion
• Summarize the essential findings and compare the case report with the literature.
• Literature should be relevant to the topic.
Conclusion
• State the lessons that may be learnt from the case report.
References
• Limited to 15–20 recent ones in Vancouver style.

NOTES